Palliative and End of Life Care for Children and Young People

Home, Hospice and Hospital

Palliative and End of Life Care for Children and Young People

Home, Hospice and Hospital

Anne Grinyer

WILEY-BLACKWELL

A John Wiley & Sons, Ltd., Publication

This edition first published 2012
© 2012 by John Wiley & Sons, Ltd.

Wiley-Blackwell is an imprint of John Wiley & Sons, formed by the merger of Wiley's global Scientific, Technical and Medical business with Blackwell Publishing.

Registered Office
John Wiley & Sons, Ltd, The Atrium, Southern Gate, Chichester, West Sussex, PO19 8SQ, UK

Editorial Offices
9600 Garsington Road, Oxford, OX4 2DQ, UK
The Atrium, Southern Gate, Chichester, West Sussex, PO19 8SQ, UK
2121 State Avenue, Ames, Iowa 50014-8300, USA

For details of our global editorial offices, for customer services and for information about how to apply for permission to reuse the copyright material in this book please see our website at www.wiley.com/wiley-blackwell.

The right of the author to be identified as the author of this work has been asserted in accordance with the UK Copyright, Designs and Patents Act 1988.

Library of Congress Cataloging-in-Publication Data

Grinyer, Anne, 1950–
   Palliative and end of life care for children and young people : home, hospice, and hospital / Anne Grinyer.
      p. ; cm.
   Includes bibliographical references and index.
   ISBN 978-0-470-65614-3 (pbk. : alk. paper)
   I. Title.
[DNLM: 1. Palliative Care. 2. Terminal Care. 3. Adolescent. 4. Child.
5. Continuity of Patient Care. 6. Hospice Care. 7. Young Adult. WS 200]
   616.02'9-dc23
                                                      2011038020

A catalogue record for this book is available from the British Library.

Wiley also publishes its books in a variety of electronic formats. Some content that appears in print may not be available in electronic books.

Set in 9/12.5pt Interstate Light by SPi Publisher Services, Pondicherry, India
Printed and bound in Malaysia by Vivar Printing Sdn Bhd

1 2012

This book is dedicated to the memory of all the young people whose stories are told in its pages, to their families who shared those stories and to the professionals who care for them. It is also dedicated to the memory of George Easton who died at the age of 23 and to his parents Helen and Geoff. Helen and Geoff's vision and commitment has supported 11 years of research and touched the lives of countless people.

Contents

Participants

Sources of original data

Hospice service evaluation: interview participants and their children

Brenda
the mother of Matthew 18 with Miller-Dieker disorder, and his sister **Katie**

Diane and **Len**
foster parents of a number of children with complex and life-limiting conditions including: Daisy aged 7 with phenoketonuria; David who died at 2 of kidney disease; Delia aged 21 with kidney disease; Ruth aged 27 with a chromosomal abnormality; Tamwar with cerebral palsy who died of a twisted bowel; Kevin aged 6 with foetal alcohol syndrome

Mandy
the mother of **Martha** 8 with Nieman-Pick Type C, and her grandmother **Elizabeth**

Melissa and **Darren**
the parents of Hannah 4 with Dravet's syndrome, and her brother **Eddie**

Lily
the mother of Karen 21 with cerebral palsy, epilepsy and scoliosis, and her sister **Martine**

Nadia and **Tony**
the foster parents of Karl 14 with cerebral palsy

Nancy
the mother of **Tess** 21 with Rett's syndrome, and her paid carer **Rory**

Susan
the mother of Bert 10 months with cerebral palsy, epilepsy and dystonia, and his grandmother **Nora** and brother **Sam**

Sharon
the mother of Edward 18 with a chromosomal disorder

The participants are in bold.

Tania
the mother of Dan who died at 16 from an unspecified neurological condition, and his sister **Ursula**

Una
the legal guardian of **Leo** 12 with chromosome deletion 6

Participants in the TYA research

Interviews

Parents and other family members

Ann
whose daughter Ellen died from bowel cancer at 23 at home

Beckie
whose daughter Billie died aged 14 from acute lymphoblastic leukaemia at home

Bianca

whose husband Ryan died 5 days before his 22 birthday from osteosarcoma at home (in his mother's house)

Candy
whose daughter Sianne died at 20 from rhabdomyosarcoma in an adult hospice

Chris
whose son Ben died aged 21 from Hodgkin's lymphoma at a local hospital

Clare
whose son Joe died aged 20 from anaplastic astrocytoma at home

Helen
whose son Simon, having travelled from Australia to London, died aged 19 from a kidney tumour in an adult hospice

Joan
whose son Stuart died in hospital from Ewing's sarcoma 3 days before his 18th birthday

Jonno and Rosie
whose son Hugh died aged 19 from Ewing's sarcoma at home at home under hospice care

Karen
whose son Mason died aged 13 from rhabdomyosarcoma at home

Laura and Arthur
whose son Ian died aged 23 from oesophageal cancer in the USA at home under hospice care

Pam and Nick
whose daughter Amy died aged 13 from acute lymphoblastic leukaemia in hospital

Pat
whose daughter Sarah died aged 26 from a desmoplastic small round intra-abdominal blue cell tumour in her marital home in Canada

Steve, Jenny and Marika
whose son (and brother) Darren died from Ewing's sarcoma aged 18 in a specialist cancer unit

Sue
whose son Alex died from osteosarcoma at the age of 22 at home in Germany

Val and Malcolm
whose son Martin died of Ewing's sarcoma at the age of 17 at home

Plus: 14 members of a bereavement group run by the Teenage Cancer Trust

Professionals

Alison
Lead cancer nurse at a district general hospital

Anne
Palliative nurse specialist in the community

Cherie
Lead clinician at an adult hospice

Chief Executive of an adult hospice (anonymous)

Clare
Director of Clinical Services at a children's hospice

Clive
General Manager of an adult hospice

Elaine
Head of Clinical Services at a children's hospice

Gill
Clinical Services Co-ordinator for Long Term Conditions in community nursing

Jenny
Tutor in Palliative Care at an adult hospice

John
Ward Manager for paediatric inpatient services at a district general hospital

Liz
Head of Care at Douglas House Hospice for young adults (16-35)

Ozzie
Professor of Adolescent Oncology

Rosemarie
Senior Palliative Care Nurse Specialist at an adult hospice with the adult home care team

Sarah
Director of Nursing at an adolescent hospice

Saul
Director of Day and Out Patient Services at an adult hospice

Sheila
Head of Care for a children's/adolescent hospice

Stella
Director of Inpatient Services at an adult hospice

Sue
TCT Programme Manager

Sue B
Clinical Nurse Manager at an adult hospice

Vikky
TCT Nurse Consultant

Wendy
Clinical Lead for Paediatric Inpatient services at a district general hospital

Teenage Cancer Trust, teenage and young adult palliative and end of life care service evaluation participants:

A total of 23 questionnaires were completed and 23 interviews were conducted with staff from seven TCT units in England, Wales and Scotland; their professions include:

- TYA Clinical Nurse Specialists
- Senior Ward Sisters
- Staff Nurses
- Consultant in Paediatric Oncology and Palliative Care Lead
- POONs nurses (Paediatric Oncology Outreach Nurses)
- CLIC Sargent Social Workers
- TYA Clinical Lead Nurses
- Lead for County Cancer Network, Palliative Care Team Leader/ Consultant in Palliative Medicine
- Activities Coordinators
- Occupational Therapists
- TCT Professional Nursing Lead and Development Manager
- Head TCT Nurse/Ward Manager
- Children and Young People's Macmillan Clinical Nurse Specialist for Outreach and Symptom Care

Additional Service Evaluation Questionnaires generated responses from 12 care settings

Foreword

Anne Grinyer's research is always compelling and absorbing. This book is no exception. It is, in essence, structured research through storytelling, making it a literary journey for the reader where the experiences of patients, friends and family are never out of focus.

Anne's contribution to our understanding of the needs of young people with cancer has been unparalleled and without her extraordinary insights, our services would be that much poorer. Palliative care and end of life support for young people is sadly an inconsistently met need but with Anne's guidance we should be able to put that right.

Simon Davies
Chief Executive Officer
Teenage Cancer Trust

Preface

This book represents the culmination of an 11-year research project, supported and funded by the George Easton Memorial Trust, during which I have examined the experiences and needs of young people with life-threatening illness (e.g. Grinyer 2002a, 2004, 2006, 2007, 2007a, 2007b, 2009). Throughout the project, age and life stage have been demonstrated as crucial factors to both the young person with the illness and to their families. During the treatment period the difficulty in finding an appropriate setting of care, the management of family relationships and the impact on family dynamics have all presented difficulties to the young person, their family and to the professionals involved in their care. What has also become apparent throughout the research findings presented in this book is that these issues are exacerbated at the end of life and need to be understood better if appropriate palliative and end of life care is to be provided.

Although the previous phases of my research have focused largely on teenagers and young adults, the scope of this book has been extended to include younger children. The boundaries between childhood, adolescence and young adulthood are often difficult to draw - indeed, this is one of the issues facing professionals when treating young people who fall between categories and services. Additionally, although my previous research has focused solely on cancer, this book includes other life-threatening and life-limiting conditions. This results not only from a need to know how palliative and end of life care is offered to and experienced by children and young people with other conditions it also allows some comparisons to be made between children who have experienced lifelong illness and those diagnosed in adolescence. This can help clarify the implications for the coordination and delivery of services to meet the needs of both cohorts.

The book provides a series of in-depth, firsthand accounts from parents whose sons and daughters have been diagnosed with life-limiting and life-threatening conditions about what it is like to care for them. In addition, interviews with the health professionals who look after children and young people in need of palliative and end of life care provide the basis for understanding the challenges they face not only in delivering care but in coordinating and collaborating with other services and meeting the needs of the young people and their families. It is to be hoped that the resulting text will be helpful to all those caring for children and young adults with life-threatening and life-limiting illness by helping parents to navigate their way through what can sometimes be a confusing array of services and to lessen feelings of isolation. It is also intended that it will assist professionals in understanding the experience for the young person and their family both during the period of care but in addition after bereavement.

Anne Grinyer

Acknowledgements

This volume could not have been produced without the help, support, encouragement and input of many people. My thanks go to Professor Sheila Payne and Zephyrine Barbarachild for their work with me on the evaluation of children's hospice services, to Zephyrine Barbarachild for her contribution to the Teenage Cancer Trust evaluation of palliative and end of life care services, to the North West Cancer Intelligence Service for their help with gathering statistical data and to Teenage Cancer Trust who assisted me in the recruitment process and who allowed me to use the palliative and end of life care evaluation data for this book. Thank you to Anthony Greenwood for his technical support; to Karen Whitcomb for her commitment to the project continuing her transcriptions even after moving to the other side of the world; to all those who painstakingly read the manuscript in advance of publication, Judith, Helen, Geoff, Jane, Julie, Jennifer and Pat and to Zephyrine for her excellent proof reading. I am grateful to The George Easton Memorial Trust for their continued support across 11 years of research and to all those who contribute to the Trust financially. However, my main thanks go to all those participants whose testimonies are at the heart of the book; to the health professionals who shared their time and wisdom with me and who introduced me to bereaved families, and finally my heartfelt thanks go to the family members who shared their stories with me and trusted me with their most painful memories.

Abbreviations

CNS   Community Nursing Service
CQC   Care Quality Commission
DGH   District General Hospital
DH   Department of Health
DMD   Duchenne Muscular Dystrophy
DNR   Do Not Resuscitate
EAPC   European Association of Palliative Care
GP   General Practitioner
ICU   Intensive Care Unit
LACS   Local Authority Children's Services
LOD   Location of Death
MDT   Multidisciplinary Team
NCIN   National Cancer Intelligence Network
NWCIS   North West Cancer Intelligence Service
PATCH   Paediatric Palliative Advice for Care at Home, Hospice or Hospital
PCT   Palliative Care Team
PCT   Primary Care Trust
POONS   Paediatric Oncology Outreach Nurses
PTC   Primary Treatment Centre
SPCU   Specialist Palliative Care Unit
TCT   Teenage Cancer Trust
TYAs   Teenagers and Young Adults
UKCCSG   United Kingdom Children's Cancer Study Group
UREC   University Research Ethics Committee
WHO   World Health Organization

Chapter 1
Palliative and End of Life Care for Children and Young Adults

The death of a child at any age and from any cause runs against the natural order (Milo 1997); indeed there is something profoundly 'wrong' about a child predeceasing its parents. As Sourkes (1977: 65) argues, the 'assumed sequence' is thrown out of order; parents who would have expected their children to care for them at the end of life instead find themselves witnessing the 'tragic absurdity' of watching their child die.

Although across the world incurable illnesses claim the lives of children on a daily basis, the culture of modern Western society tends to 'push awareness of these personal tragedies to the back of our minds' (Riches and Dawson 2000: 9). Death and illness are hidden from view in a society where most acute illness and the majority of deaths are managed out of sight in hospitals and hospices. As a result, family members engaged actively on a daily basis with the care of a child with life-threatening or life-limiting illness can feel isolated in a world hidden from view. Their struggles may remain unobserved and they can find it difficult to access the support needed for the child, siblings and their own welfare.

Benini et al. (2008) define 'life-limiting' conditions as those where a premature death is usual and these would include such conditions as Duchenne muscular dystrophy (DMD) and a variety of chromosomal disorders. However, although a 'life-threatening illness' carries a high risk of premature death, there is also a chance of the illness being cured and it is usually this term that is applied to cancer diagnoses. According to ACT (2011a), there are at any given time more than 23,000 children with life-limiting or life-threatening illness in the UK, half of whom will have substantial palliative care needs. Approximately 80,000-100,000 family members and carers are involved in the support of these children, whose needs may be complex; thus, in the UK alone there are significant numbers of individuals with the potential to feel alone and isolated. Indeed, almost by definition, the families caring for a child with complex and life-limiting health problems are likely to become socially isolated as a result.

Runswick-Cole (2010: 813) claims that services for children with life-limiting illnesses have been poor, but there has been little research in this area because of what she calls the 'wider social embarrassment' of talking about death and the need to distance disability from the 'tragedy stories' of the past. Her findings suggest that families experience both social isolation and poverty, lack appropriate support and worry about the costs of care. However, the recent increasing recognition of the challenges faced by both families and professionals caring for a dying child has resulted in a number of policy documents and academic texts – many of which are cited here. What this book adds to a growing body of literature is the voices of the people charged with the care of children, teenagers and young adults whose lives are coming to an end. The following chapters draw upon in-depth interviews with both professionals and family members in order to understand what it is like to care for a child who will die.

The topic of palliative and end of life care for children and young adults is so wide that some boundaries have had to be drawn to structure both the data collection and the remit of this text. Consequently, the book is based mainly on data derived from two studies, one looking at the specific issues relating to cancer in teenagers and young adults, the other an evaluation of children's hospice services. The contrasting experiences of the two cohorts results in some fundamental differences in the nature of the data collected. The use of health care services, the type of services used, the length of time care may be palliative and the transition between palliative and end of life care, may vary considerably according to the type of condition with which a child is diagnosed. This means that the empirical chapters that focus on a particular health care setting reveal very different types of experience and usage within that setting. Not all issues will be relevant to both cohorts, but the contrast becomes part of the analysis.

It is hoped that such a comparison will be beneficial for those planning services by answering such questions as: what are the similarities and differences between children born with a life-limiting condition and young people diagnosed with acute life-threatening illness in adolescence? When do services need to be separate? What are the contrasts in the families' experiences and needs? In addition, drawing on the accounts of both professionals and families allows the perspectives of each to be heard, and for the complex dynamic that operates in such a highly charged and often distressing context to be better understood. Quotations and case study material from in-depth interviews have been selected to provide examples that give an insight into what it is like to support children and young adults at the end of their lives. The quantity of original qualitative data that acts as the basis for this book amounts to some 400,000 words, thus it is impossible to do justice to each and every transcript, but readers can be secure in the knowledge that, through the process of analysis, the full range of experience has been represented and that claims made in the text are based on a wealth of data that remains largely unobservable. Although individual participants' stories have been selected to represent the wider data set, I have tried to remain true to the spirit of all those who participated in the research and represent the range of views, opinions and experiences.

The book begins with an overview of the literature and policy in the area and then moves on to present chapters based on the firsthand accounts of the participants. There are chapters on palliative and end of life care as it is experienced in the home, in children's, adult and adolescent hospices and in hospitals. These are followed by a chapter on how parents and professionals manage communications with the children and young people about end of life and how they negotiate the transition from curative to palliative treatment. This chapter also considers the bereavement needs of the parents, how they can best prepare themselves for their loss and how their grief and loss may be shaped by the way in which end of life decisions were made and shared – or not – with their lost children. Drawing on the analysis of the empirical data, the final chapter considers the implications for policy and practice. The appendix includes an account of the methods used to gather the original data on which the empirical chapters are based.

Defining palliative and end of life care

This book addresses both palliative and end of life care. The boundaries between the two may be blurred and some of the young people whose stories are told in this book were in receipt of palliative care while also receiving active treatment; in some cases the palliative phase was brief, in others it continued for years. It would therefore be helpful to define the terms. Clark and Wright (2003) provide a summary of the World Health Organization's (WHO) definition as follows:

> Palliative care is an approach that improves the quality of life of patients and their families facing the problems associated with life-threatening illness, through the prevention and relief of suffering by means of early identification and impeccable assessment and treatment of pain and other problems, physical, psychosocial and spiritual. Palliative care:
>
> - Provides relief from pain and other distressing symptoms
> - Affirms life and regards dying as a normal process
> - Intends neither to hasten nor postpone death
> - Integrates the psychological and spiritual aspects of patient care
> - Offers a support system to help patients live as actively as possible until death
> - Offers a support system to help the family cope during the patient's illness and in their own bereavement
> - Uses a team approach to address the needs of patients and their families, including bereavement counselling, if indicated
> - Will enhance quality of life, and may also positively influence the course of the illness
> - Is applicable early in the course of the illness, in conjunction with other therapies that are intended to prolong life, such as chemotherapy or radiation therapy, and includes those investigations needed to better understand and manage distressing clinical complications.
>
> (Clark and Wright 2003: 1-2)

This definition makes it clear that palliative care may mean 'end of life care' but can also be used in conjunction with active treatments that may prolong life and can be utilised as a strategy early in an illness to relieve suffering. In a slightly different use of terminology Benini et al. (2008) say that although terminal care is not the same as palliative care, palliative care can include terminal care; this distinction they say is crucial as it can establish eligibility criteria in a field where they claim that a minority of children across Europe benefit from palliative care.

The definition of end of life care offered by Kirsti and Dyer (2006) suggests that the precise definition of 'end of life' is problematic:

> There is no exact definition of end of life; however, research supports the following components:
>
> 1. The presence of a chronic disease(s) or symptoms or functional impairments that persist but may also fluctuate; and
> 2. The symptoms or impairments resulting from the underlying irreversible disease that require formal either paid, professional or informal unpaid or volunteer care and can lead to death.
>
> **End of Life Care**
> *End of Life Care* is the care provided to a person in their final stages of life. Also known as hospice care, comfort care, supportive care, palliative care or symptom management.
> (Kirsti and Dyer 2006)

So it seems from this definition that 'palliative care' has been subsumed into 'end of life care'. Field and Behrman (2003: 34) suggest that 'end of life care' has no precise meaning but is used to describe the care that focuses on the preparation for a death that is anticipated. Field and Behrman also say that, together, palliative and end of life care should promote clear and culturally sensitive communication in order to help patients and families understand the diagnosis, prognosis and treatment options available.

Challenges to the delivery of palliative and end of life care for children and young people

This book addresses issues of both palliative and end of life care, thus it encompasses the care that may be given to children and young people with life-threatening and life-limiting illness perhaps for some considerable time before the end of their lives. This is particularly true of the children and young people who have been born with or develop a chronic condition in early childhood. They may in fact use palliative care services for the whole of their lives, whereas, in contrast, the teenagers and young adults (TYAs) diagnosed with cancer will undergo an intensive phase of treatment with the aim of cure. For those TYAs diagnosed with cancer who are not cured, their period of palliative care may be much shorter and raise different issues and challenges.

The European Association of Palliative Care (EAPC 2009) states that although access to palliative care for adults with incurable conditions is regarded as a right, the provision for those in the paediatric age group is still in its early stages and services for children and their families are fragmented and inconsistent. The reasons given for this are that the numbers of eligible children are fewer in comparison to adults, there can be a gap in organisational and managerial policy, a shortage of competent medical staff and cultural issues relating to the care of dying children that affect social acceptance. This is echoed by Price and McFarlane (2009) who say that difficulties arise from the differing needs of children and families, the variation in the availability of services and a lack of understanding by policy makers as to what constitutes palliative care.

Benini et al. (2008) also suggest that symptom management at the end of a child's life can be inadequate and that, along with clinical problems, the psychological, social and spiritual aspects may receive inadequate attention. These authors suggest this is a global problem, that insufficient resources are dedicated to this area of medicine and geographical location may affect access as may disease type.

The Department of Health (DH) policy document 'Better Care: Better Lives' (2008) identifies a number of challenges to the delivery of palliative care for children including:

- The change in the profile of children with life-limiting or life-threatening conditions over the last 20 years due to technological advances and increased survival rates of low-birthweight babies
- Poor co-ordination of services across the statutory and voluntary sectors, particularly transition between children's and adult services
- Little acknowledgement of the need for earlier interventions and assessments
- Insufficient investment in local prevention strategies or timely referral to specialist services
- High thresholds/eligibility criteria for accessing existing palliative care services
- Insufficient prioritisation for children with life-limiting or life-threatening conditions, and short term funding
- Lack of transparency/agreement between budget holders about who will fund which aspect of care and support
- Lack of capability, capacity and equity within universal services to meet many of the needs of these children (and related workforce issues, including shortage of specialist staff)
- Lack of information, consultation and empowerment for children with life-limiting or life-threatening conditions and their families
- The need for a range of specialist short breaks which would include breaks in the home, in children's hospices and the other voluntary sector providers, as well as better co-ordinated specialist support.
  (DH 2008: 15-16)

Thus, it can be seen that although there is recognition of the increasing need for children's palliative care services, there are a number of problems associated with its widespread provision and its availability to all children and families in need of such support.

In order to address the issues raised above and to provide high-quality services to children with life-threatening and life-limiting conditions and their families, the DH (2008) state that palliative care should form a thread throughout the lives of these children and that palliative care needs to be high on the agenda of those responsible for the provision of children's services. To achieve this, the DH identified eight strategic development goals, which are:

- Improved data
- Equality of access to universal services
- Responsible and accountable leadership
- Choice in preferred place of care and expansion of community services
- Better end of life care
- Stronger commissioning and value for money
- Successful transition between children's and adult services
- Planning and developing an effective and responsive workforce
  (DH 2008: 18)

The needs of families and children include physical, psychological, social and spiritual care, and the Department of Health policy document 'Better Care: Better Lives' (2008) recognises that families who have the responsibility of caring for a child with life-limiting and complex conditions need to be supported. The report also recognises that families need a more personal, community-based service where agencies work together. Continuity of care is also important so that in times of crisis the professionals caring for their child are known and trusted.

Settings of care

As Brook et al. (2006: 533) argue, the palliative care journey from diagnosis through to bereavement, presents many problems. If the primary objective is to support the child and family, the care provided should be tailored to their needs. However, flexibility is necessary as these needs can change over time; the birth of a new baby, the illness of a sibling perhaps from the same condition, bereavement, divorce and other life events can all affect the provision of care.

Bearing in mind these changing needs, there are a number of settings in which care can be delivered. Many young people will be cared for in their homes for much of the time. This, Brook et al. argue, can reduce the disruption to family life, be beneficial to siblings and may be the preference of the sick child. Similarly Hynson (2006) reports that many families describe home care as positive, subject as it is to fewer interruptions and intrusions. Feudtner et al. (2007) claim that since 1989, children with complex, chronic conditions are increasingly dying at home as a result of evolving epidemiology, advances in home-based medical technology and changes in attitudes. Nevertheless, end of life care at home can present challenges and Hynson reminds us that it is not desirable for all families. But even those families who choose to support end of life care at home may be ill-prepared for the demands; as Contro and Scofield say (2006), they can be required to perform care-giving tasks they had not anticipated. These issues and experiences are addressed through the firsthand accounts in Chapter 2. Home-based outreach care provided by hospices is also considered in this chapter on home deaths rather than being included in the chapter on hospice deaths.

Chapter 3 examines the difficulties of providing hospice care. In the UK 'hospice care' is taken to mean care within a hospice building, whereas in the USA it has a different meaning and encompasses a philosophy of care that is usually delivered in the home rather than in an inpatient facility and the term can be used to cover all palliative care (Brook et al. 2006: 542). This book uses the UK interpretation of hospice care. Brook et al. establish that only 20% of children who use hospice care die in a hospice, although they can be transferred from a hospital for hospice care when the end of life approaches. The challenge for hospices in providing care – particularly transitional care – is addressed in Chapter 3, in which the differing roles of paediatric, adolescent and adult hospices are considered through accounts from both families and professionals.

Children's end of life care may also take place in hospital, indeed the majority of all child deaths in the UK and the USA occur in hospital (Brook et al. 2006: 542). Of these deaths 60% are due to complex, chronic life-limiting conditions. Although the majority of childhood cancer deaths occur in the home – Brook et al. cite UKCCSG figures of 78% – where the death is a result of the complications of curative treatment, these deaths tend to take place in hospital. The majority of children who die in hospital do so on a paediatric intensive care unit (ICU). Brook et al. (2006: 541–542) claim that much can be done to establish a 'home from home' environment in hospital. In addition, the provision of shared care between a primary treatment centre (PTC) and a local hospital can allow a child to be treated nearer to home and where this is not possible family accommodation may be provided. Yet, according to these authors, families continue to report 'confusing, inadequate or uncaring communication' and feel that they have lost control. The bereaved families of children who have died from cancer in hospital also report greater guilt, anxiety and depression than those whose children die at home. The experience of hospital deaths is considered in Chapter 4; however, many of the empirical examples in this chapter relate to young adults with cancer whose hospital care at the end of life can be particularly complicated to organise.

Transition from paediatric to adult care

The age range covered in this book is wide, including children, teenagers and young adults. Thus, the age band encompasses the transitional stage between paediatric and adult services when, as a result of their age, young people may find themselves cared for in inappropriate environments. As more young people are surviving life-threatening and life-limiting illnesses into adulthood they need to make the move from children's services to adult services (DH 2008, Marsh et al. 2011). However, a seamless transition is difficult to achieve if there is a gap between services that results in the young person remaining too long in an unsuitable paediatric environment or being transferred too soon into an adult care setting with older people. Where close relationships with paediatric staff have been developed both by the young people and their families, the move can seem a particularly daunting prospect. Thus, successful transition from children's to adult care involves careful planning in order to ensure a seamless process. To achieve this, the DH (2008) suggests that it is important to:

- start early
- be flexible
- be individually tailored to meet the needs of the young person and their family
- continue, if necessary, following the transfer to adult care
  (DH 2008: 40)

The co-ordination of transition is crucial and a key/named worker or lead worker should in ideal circumstances be identified to oversee the process (DH 2008). This should ensure links between the services. The Association of Children's Palliative Care (ACT) Transition Care Pathway provides a framework (2007). ACT acknowledges that there is a wide variation of services across the country but identifies key principles for the move to be successfully managed. These include for young people:

- specific service provision
- development of skills of self-management and self-determination
- supported psychosocial development
- involvement of young people
- peer involvement
- support for changed relationships with parents/carers
- provision of choice
- provision of information
- focus on the young person's strengths for future development

For parents:

- support for adjustment to changed relationships with young people
- parental involvement in service planning
- a family-centred approach
- provision of information
  (Association of Children's Palliative Care 2007: 10)

The documents cited provide a framework for the provision of palliative care for children and young people, and their recommendations act as a useful context for the consideration of service provision for the age group. However, they suggest that although the need for appropriate services has been recognised as an issue of significance, there is currently inconsistent provision. Craig (2006) argues that it can be difficult to identify the most appropriate team to take on the care of an adolescent and that in addition paediatricians may be reluctant to let go of their patients and allow them to move to adult services.

The problems of transition are summarised by the subtitle of a Report on the issue prepared by Marsh et al. (2011): *Small numbers, huge needs, cruel and arbitrary division of services*. Marsh et al. (2011: 6) argue that 'there is **no clear model** of care underpinning services' and that professionals:

> **live in silos**, locked into separate and differing assumptions, structurally separated systems that are Children's and Adult services ... **have few means of sharing insights into each other's work** and culture and find it difficult to identify and adopt good practice ... **struggle to operate transition planning procedures** ... and 'work around' dysfunctional systems. (Original emphasis)
> (Marsh et al. 2011: 6)

Marsh et al. claim that young people's experience of transition is poor both in terms of the services provision and their level of autonomy. Parents too, according to these authors, have a poor experience in terms of the impact on their son or daughter and on themselves as there may be fewer opportunities for respite care. Suggestions for how the system could be improved include:

- a **broader support system**, taking on the social issues raised by young people
- a continuing **clear clinical lead** role
- **cross system networks**
- **young person-centred** ethos
- **joint** training and development
  (Marsh et al. 2011: 8, original emphasis)

These transitional issues and the extent to which the recommendations made by Marsh et al. are already recognised or in place, are addressed throughout the book.

Children and young adults with cancer and place of death

Despite the wide range of illness from which children and young people die, neoplasms are the main medical cause of death for 1-24-year-olds (National Cancer Intelligence Network 2011), thus it is important that we have some notion

Table 1.1 Descriptive statistics for cancer deaths registered in England and Wales in 1995–9 for children and adolescents (age range 0–15) and young adults (age range 16–24). Values are numbers (percentages) unless otherwise indicated.

Place of death	Children and adolescents (0-15 years, n=1725)	Young adults (16-24 years, n=1472)
General hospital or multifunction site	43	58
Home	52	30
Hospice	3	9
Other	2	3

Extract from Higginson and Thompson (2003: 478). Reproduced with permission from BMJ Publishing Group Ltd.

Table 1.2 Percentage of deaths 1998–2002.

Place of death	0-13 years	14-24 years	25+ years
Hospital	28	37	33
Home	30	23	21
Hospice	7	5	8
Unknown	35	35	38

of where children and young people die from malignancies that are the biggest single case of non-accidental death. Based on an epidemiological study of 3,197 children and young people with cancer, Higginson and Thompson (2003) noted that there are a relatively high proportion of home deaths (Table 1.1).

Yet we can see that the proportion of home deaths is higher for children (52%) than for young adults (30%). Moreover, as Higginson and Thompson comment, 'This is higher than for the United States (20%) and for adults (26%)'. It is also evident that very few children or young adults died in hospices as might have been expected. The reasons for these apparent anomalies may be accounted for through the empirical data in this book and are the subject of discussion in the following chapters.

In 2010, The North West Cancer Intelligence Service (NWCIS) prepared data on place of death on [my] request. A summary of these data for the North West Region of the UK from 1998 to 2008 is given in Tables 1.2 and 1.3.

What is perhaps most surprising is the percentage of 'unknowns', where the location of death could not be identified. This means that the data have to be treated with some care. However, we can see that the figures are relatively consistent across the 10-year period, suggesting that services have not developed or changed significantly during that time. What is more important is that

Table 1.3 Percentage of deaths 2003–2008.

Place of death	0-13 years	14-24 years	25+ years
Hospital	34	40	41
Home	28	29	23
Hospice	10	6	9
Unknown	28	25	25

the percentages for the places of death for young adults (14-24 years) are in the same rank order as those reported in the Higginson and Thompson study: hospital, home, hospice.

A later briefing from the National Cancer Intelligence Network (NCIN) (2011) offers figures for place of death for children, teenagers and young adults who died from cancer in England between 2000 and 2009, during which time 2611 young people died before the age of 15 and 2975 died between the ages of 15 and 24. Although survival rates are improving, with more than 78% surviving at least 5 years after diagnosis, cancers are still the main medical cause of death for 1-24-year-olds. The NCIN figures show that of the children: 47% died in hospital, 39% in their own home, 11% in a hospice or specialist palliative care unit (SPCU) and 3% in a care home. However, for the teenagers and young adults: 52% died in a hospital, 32% in their own home 13% in a hospice or SPCU and 3% in a care home. Again, we have the same rank order for place of death.

The NCIN study shows that deaths from leukaemia or lymphoma were more likely to take place in hospital, whereas the patients who died in a hospice or SPCU were more likely have bone tumours and soft tissue sarcomas, although the highest proportion dying in their own homes had bone tumours. The data also suggest that place of death was more likely to be in a hospital for Asian patients than for White patients. In summary, children were less likely to die in hospital than teenagers or young adults, and ethnicity and socio-demographics are also likely to have influenced place of death.

Although statistics on place of death give us some idea of where children and young people with cancer die, we can gather little about how – or even if – a choice was made or what the experience was like. However, there are a few studies that address the more qualitative issues surrounding end of life care and place of death. For example, according to Contro et al. (2002), families tend to be dissatisfied with communication with health professionals at the end of life and feel that their wishes are disregarded. Montel et al. (2009) argue that such communication difficulties with health professionals or within the family are factors that are likely to interfere with choice of place of care at the end of life.

The first study on place of death for young adults with cancer in France was carried out by Montel et al. (2009), who claim that theirs is also the first study to examine the factors that influence the choice of place of death in this age group with cancer. As these authors say, it is essential to carry out such research in order to meet the needs of the young patients and their families at the end of life. Of the 21 young people in the study, 19 died in hospital and only two at home. Montel et al. attempted to identify the determinants of choice of the place of death. Ninety per cent of the families said that they had not felt that they actually 'chose' the place of death, but would nevertheless have chosen the hospital where the death did in fact take place, had they had a choice. Thus, they were not expressing dissatisfaction with the service but with their lack of options.

Only three out of Montel et al.'s sample of 21 were informed about the palliative care mobile unit, but were as a consequence enabled to support a home death. Nine of the sample were given information about the existence of home hospitalisation. Motivations for the 'choices' made were, according to Montel et al., as follows. There is a desire to keep the child at home for as long as possible to retain normality and to be surrounded by family and friends, and most of the young people wished to stay at home for as long as possible. However, some parents felt that home care signalled the end of curative treatment and thus confirmed the approaching death of their son or daughter. Others believed they would have to leave a home where their child had died as the memories would be too painful and that the medical invasion of their home would be a negative experience. The protection of siblings from proximity to the death was also an issue.

The choices available to families and young people about place of death is a theme that runs throughout this book for both the TYAs with cancer and the children with other complex and life-limiting conditions.

Preparation for bereavement and bereavement support

The bereavement support after a child's death is, according to Lenton et al. (2006), an integral part of palliative care. Lewis and Prescott (2006) also claim that such support should be available at whatever age a child dies under whatever circumstances and in whatever setting. There should be a range of flexible and sensitive services that extend to the wider family if necessary as well as to the dying child. Preparation for bereavement is also an essential part of this process as Contro and Scofield (2006) state, most parents say they would have benefited from more preparatory information.

However, although preparatory information may be important, so too is an element of control at the end of life in terms of preparing for how and where the death will take place. Dussel et al. (2009) undertook a study of 140 bereaved parents of children between 1 and 10 years old in the USA, and discovered the longer term effects of having the opportunity to plan the place of death. This study found that in those cases where the treatment options had been explained clearly at the end of life, there was a greater likelihood of planning for place of death. Ninety-seven per cent of the parents who planned their child's location of death also reported that their child had actually died in their chosen setting.

Planning was also associated with parents feeling more prepared for the death, experiencing less invasive care and having fewer regrets after the death. Dussel et al. suggest that experiences at the time of death have a lasting effect and that planning may affect long-term bereavement outcomes. According to these authors, although death at home might be preferred by many, the actual location of death (LOD) may be less important than is assumed, as, among the attributes of a good death, dying at home was the least important. These authors acknowledge that their sample was mainly white and middle class and suggest that there may be ethnic and racial differences.

Even when the death of a child has been expected, the actual death is still profoundly shocking, an unparalleled agony likened to an amputation (Thomas and Chalmers 2009). According to these authors, poor bereavement care can exacerbate and prolong families' distress, whereas sensitive and appropriate care can help families grieve; they too emphasise the need for bereavement care to be an integral part of palliative care.

Thomas and Chalmers (2009) argue that there is a need for professionals to examine their own beliefs and values relating to death and dying, yet it is also important to remember that when planning bereavement services and support, the culture and ethnicity of the families need to be taken into account. Brown (2006) argues that ethnicity and culture profoundly influence how families experience death. She claims that over the last two decades there has been an increasing awareness of the importance of listening to parents and of the need to avoid stereotypes concerning the level and nature of support that would be welcomed by families. Thus, information about different faiths and cultures is only relevant if it is meaningful to the families concerned. Although this book does not include examples of deaths in families from ethnic minorities, Brown's claim that families need to be heard and responded to on an individual basis that is meaningful to them is still very relevant, as there can be a tendency to implement a model of grief as the basis for post-bereavement services without taking into account the individual and differing needs of families. These issues are addressed in Chapter 5.

Summary

So what do we know about how and where young people die? It is clear that there is a great deal of literature on the topic and a number of policy documents that address many of the issues and difficulties. Yet there is still much that remains unknown as the statistical data provide a restricted understanding of the experience. As Benini et al. (2008) say, there are no published data on the incidence of life-limiting and life-threatening illness in children for most countries in Europe. Even where there is information on service provision that includes statistics on hospital, home and hospice deaths, this nevertheless tells us little about what choices were offered and raises the following questions. Did the setting of palliative and end of life care and place of death reflect the families' and children's wishes and preferences, or was there no option? How were those settings experienced? Has the increasing recognition of the challenges of transition translated into improved services? Were professionals and parents able to discuss their child's death with them in advance? These questions are addressed in the remainder of this book, drawing primarily on research with health professionals, parents and some children who use the services. Through their accounts we can chart the challenges for service providers and the difficulties faced by the children and their families in obtaining appropriate care.

Chapter 2
Home-based Palliative and End of Life Care

Many families whose child has a life-limiting condition prefer to care for their child at home as this causes the least disruption to family life and routines (Brook et al. 2006). As Brook et al. say, children with life-limiting conditions may experience deterioration in their health over months or years, necessitating an increase in support and care. As a result, adaptations may need to be made to their homes and special equipment provided to meet the needs of their increasing physical dependency. Over the course of such deterioration in health, families – particularly in the domestic environment – need the support of a multidisciplinary team of professionals. For a child or young adult with a lifelong condition, the end of life may follow an extended period of treatment intended to prolong life, and, according to Brook et al. (2006), it may not be until the last 24–48 hours that it becomes clear that death is imminent. Although these authors suggest that both professionals and families may be reluctant to acknowledge that death is approaching, decisions need to be made in advance in order to provide appropriate end of life care. Brook et al. note that families often want their child to die at home and say there is evidence to suggest that outcomes are better if this is the case (Brook et al. 2006: 535). They do not specify what these 'outcomes' are and clearly, as it is not the survival of the child, the implication is that there are benefits for the family in the grieving process. Although Feudtner et al. (2007) claim that home deaths are increasing for children; they also acknowledge that racial and ethnic disparities may influence the likelihood of a home death.

Brook et al. (2006) emphasise the importance of both the family and the child being involved in decisions about end of life care and that honest and comprehensive information must be given if a home death is chosen so that all those involved understand what they are taking on. These authors acknowledge that the level of support can vary markedly from one family to another, and a family may have little idea of how much support they will need. Families from ethnic minorities may, however, be reluctant to ask for help, leading professionals perhaps to assume that their community is providing support. However, as Brook et al. say, this assumption may be incorrect. Although the demands on families are great in supporting a home death,

Palliative and End of Life Care for Children and Young People: Home, Hospice and Hospital, First Edition. Anne Grinyer.

Hynson (2006) argues that for some home care can be very positive and allows children and parents to feel more in control of the process. There are fewer interruptions and intrusions, siblings have their needs attended to more easily, and friends and family may be more accessible.

Thus far the discussion has focused on children with long-term life-limiting conditions. For children and young people with cancer the situation historically has been different, and home care has developed from a particular context (Lenton et al. 2006). Although these authors acknowledge that specialist cancer services were among the first to recognise the need for palliative care, the majority of such services were hospital-based in oncology units and reliant on specialist nurses. Nevertheless, Davis (2009) suggests that although there is a general assumption that children and young people with malignancies are more likely to have the choice to die at home, this is not necessarily the case. She cites figures that show that between 1995 and 1999 only 52% of children and 30% of young people with cancer died at home, and that being from a lower social class or living in a deprived area reduced the likelihood of a home death. However, Davis claims that since the 1980s an increasing number of children with malignancies have been able to die at home because of the paediatric oncology outreach nurses (POONS) attached to regional oncology centres. Davis argues, however, that children with other conditions do not have this option, thus reducing their chance of a home death. Davis cites a 2004 House of Commons Report, which acknowledges that not only is the likelihood of a home death associated with a child's condition, it is also geographically dependent.

Services for children with cancer are, according to Vickers et al. (2007), well supported by POONS alongside general practitioners (GPs), noting:

> It might be anticipated that, as the child's condition deteriorates and the end of life approaches, families would lose confidence in their ability to care for the child at home. In our study, the reverse was true. During the final month, the proportion of families preferring home had risen to 80%. This suggests that families felt empowered by the support given to them by the POONS, supported in turn by the oncologist and GP and respective tertiary and community teams.
>
> The palliative needs of children with cancer are different from those with other life-limiting conditions, and it has been suggested that children's hospices may not be suitable locations. Most oncology centres in the UK have an infrastructure in place for such children to be cared for at home. In this study, only a small number of children dying with cancer were reported to have spent time in a children's hospice. They may represent a more important resource in the future, as their working links with oncology units become closer.
> (Vickers et al. 2007: 4475)

It is important to remember that although much of the literature suggests that a home death is desirable, and that outcomes are more positive and it is what families and children want, not all families can support such an option. Davis (2009) cites Dominica (1987) as follows:

> While home may be regarded as the most appropriate environment for care, this may not be possible or even desirable for some families. There may, as Dominica (1987) has observed, be unwillingness by parents to want to live in a house where their child has died ... Understandably, some parents may feel totally overwhelmed by caring for their dying child alongside other family and home responsibilities. This may be particularly difficult for single parents, who have to bear the care of their dying child alone and unsupported.
> (Davis 2009: 174)

So the chances of a home death may be shaped by a number of factors: the child's condition, the availability of services, ethnicity, and the social and financial resources of the family and parents. We now move to the empirical data to examine how these issues are experienced by families managing a home death for either a child with complex life-limiting conditions or a teenager or young adult with cancer. In the case of home-based care there may be a number of providers, hospices being one of several sources of such support. Because this chapter and the following two are organised around the setting of care – in this case the home – rather than the care provider, I have included the outreach services delivered by hospices in this chapter on home-based care rather than the following chapter on hospice care.

Findings

The quality and extent of outreach provision in the home for children with complex and life-limiting conditions

This chapter begins its analysis of the empirical data by examining the issues relating to care in the home for families using a children's hospice service. Unlike young adults who are diagnosed with cancer unexpectedly during early adulthood, children and young people with long-term life-limiting conditions are likely to have received home-based care for much of their lives. At the end of their lives, because the care they receive at home may be an extension of the support to which they and their families have become accustomed, adaptations may already have been made to the family house, equipment provided and sources of support identified and put in place. It may also be the case that what is understood by professionals as 'end of life care' for those diagnosed with complex and life-limiting conditions, is experienced by the families and young people as a continuation of the home-based care already in place. As Brook et al. (2006) say, it may not be until 24 hours prior to death that the 'palliative care' is identified as 'end of life care', so in the discussion that follows for this cohort the demarcation between palliative and end of life care may be blurred.

Anne, a palliative nurse specialist in the community, reiterated the problem of identifying when 'end of life' care begins:

> I think the main challenge is about when is end of life, because ... with younger people they do bounce back. And I think the challenge is, with younger people you can't always gauge when that time is when they're going to die. Yes, you have an idea that they're what we call 'in the dying phase', but to know when they're imminently dying is quite difficult, because they're like small children, they bounce up and down. And you know what you see one day is not how you see the next. So usually the challenge is, we don't have as much time for preparation as we would do for somebody in the older age group.
> (Anne)

This is, of course, the case whatever the care setting, however, when the care is home-based there can be a slippage from palliative care into end of life care, which can occur without any decision having had to be made about how that process will be managed. Indeed most of the comments on outreach or home-based care were not specifically about 'end of life', as most of the families interviewed had children still living and did not want to engage with end of life issues. As there can be an understandable resistance to engaging with end of life care issues, these were usually alluded to obliquely. However, there was much reflection on the quality and extent of home-based care that could be defined as palliative in that it relieved suffering, improved the quality of life and offered support but was not primarily 'curative', although it may have acted positively on the course of the illness (Clark and Wright 2003).

Outreach care

Despite the blurring of the boundaries between palliative and end of life care, for many of the families of the chronically sick children the care they received at home became a routine part of the support that enabled them to care for their child. The following comments, for example, were typical; suggesting that outreach care can be useful in the ongoing management of chronic conditions: '[The outreach sister] did come out for something last year, and she was really good and kept following up with calls. I can't remember what it was ... I think it was her bowels or something' (Nancy), and 'We have had the outreach service when he has not been well, or when we have been worried, but not so much of the home-care nursing; it is more for advice that we used it' (Brenda). It was clear, however, with these families that because the care that they received was not perceived to be 'end of life' care but part of ongoing supportive care, it was not valued as highly as inpatient respite care.

In these examples Brenda and Nancy were both referring to hospice outreach services, but home-based care may be delivered by a variety of services and agencies. Even those families actively supported by a hospice might receive their home-based care from different sources, such as the children's community nursing team, which can cause some confusion – who to call for what purpose – indicating a need for coordination between services. There may also be a perceived discrepancy in the quality of the different services. For certain families there was some disappointment with the 'patchy' outreach provision delivered by agency nurses.

In a paradoxical example, one family whose baby son Barnie had not been expected to live, was given an 'early' Christmas in October in anticipation of his imminent death. His care at this time took place as an inpatient at the hospice, but unexpectedly he survived the crisis and was still alive at Christmas. In contrast to their experience of the sensitive and imaginative support they were given during Barnie's inpatient stay, this family found the home-based support over the Christmas period itself 'very poor'. Outreach services were closed over the holiday weekend so Barnie had to be admitted to hospital. Although the hospice staff phoned every day and the outreach staff visited on Sundays, this situation nevertheless resulted in Barnie's first, and possibly only, Christmas being spent in hospital rather than at home because a home-based service was unavailable.

The same family were grateful for a home visit to replace a feeding tube but were told that if it happened again they should go to the hospital. The mother's comments below indicate that there had perhaps been a failure of communication about the appropriate service to contact, and when home-based care is appropriate as opposed to a hospital visit:

> When [we] had a nurse here [at home], she noticed his syringe driver had an air bubble in it. I phoned up and one of the [hospice] staff, she was just really rude, and she said 'Well it has got nothing to do with us, phone up one of the district nurses'. So I phoned up the district nurses and they were like, 'Well, the hospice has got an outreach service, we can't come and do it all the time', because I think they only work so many hours a day, don't they … ? I think they definitely do need more outreach. I got really stressed because I didn't know where to phone, and she could have been a bit nicer about it. Then when his NG tube came out … I phoned up the hospice, and then [someone] came out and more or less said she didn't get paid so don't phone her up again, sort of thing, go to [the hospital]. So they were the only two things that really annoyed me, because I am thinking you are meant to have an outreach service. I don't like to just take him up to the hospital to put a new tube down because of all the infection … if that was the case, then don't give [a staff member] an outreach call if she doesn't get paid. Fair enough, if she doesn't get paid it's not fair for her to come out, but when we have got him here …
> (Susan)

On other occasions, families were told by hospice services that for certain home-based needs they should call the district nursing team, indicating evidence of confusion over who to call for what purpose; and although hospice staff would make home visits, there was an impression that under some circumstances these might be resented. In contrast, Matthew, a young adult cared for in independent supported living, still had weekly outreach visits from the hospice as there were no nursing staff on the residential support team. This was greatly valued by his mother Brenda and demonstrates that home-based care can be extended to a 'home' that is not necessarily the family home but rather is the place of residence of the young person, the palliative support extending to end of life if necessary.

What can reasonably be expected from outreach care?

It was clear from some of the accounts given by parents of children with life-limiting illness that although outreach care in the home was valued highly, more would be welcomed, thus raising the question of how much care in the home it is reasonable to expect. Liz, the Head of Nursing at a young adult hospice attached to a children's hospice said:

> There appears to be a very heavy dependence on charity-based organisa-tions, but increasingly, charity-based organisations are saying we have to be paid something to deliver this service, because actually the statutory sector is now relying on the charities to deliver the service and therefore it is only right that the statutory services pay something towards the provision that they're making use of. So it's becoming an increasingly com-plex picture in an environment where there's less and less money available. And also, in an environment where children with increasingly complex health needs are living [longer], because we are so actively intervening, either at the stage of neonates and resuscitating profoundly disabled babies, you know, and continuing to intervene all through their young childhood. So we are now getting more and more children with very, very complex needs, and it's very expensive to support them. There's a growing population of what are termed 'technology dependent children', so chil-dren for example who are completely dependent on ventilators the whole of their lives, and can have incredibly good quality lives from their point of view and from their families' point of view, but it's very complex ... and it's very expensive to deliver care to those children. And there are not that many places yet who are going to have the staff with the skills they need to deliver the appropriate care to those children ... And so yes, whilst families do say the care that we get is absolutely fantastic, they will immediately follow that by saying but we need more of it.
> (Liz)

Liz continued by saying that the burden on families is 'massive' as many of the children need 24-hour care with some parents having to get up every hour or two throughout the night. As a result they become exhausted but the children's hospices cannot be expected to 'do it all'. However, as Liz said, most children will receive support from a variety of sources including other charitable organisations and the local children's nursing team.

Although hospice outreach care may be a very welcome option for some families, not all hospices have the capacity to provide outreach care 24 hours a day, 7 days a week, and not all families are able, either physically or emotionally, to support a home death. So although this may be a good solution in some instances, it will not always be available or acceptable. It is also essential that a family and young person planning a home death have assurance that services will be available. When I interviewed Sarah she was in the process of raising the funds to set up an adolescent hospice, which would have 10 inpatient beds for the support of patients with a variety of conditions. However, the majority of the young people would be cared for in their homes, with care services extending across a 20-mile radius from the hospice, supporting up to 50 patients and available 24 hours a day, 7 days a week. Sarah emphasised the importance of this part of the service:

> It's really, really important ... that they are able to access 24 hour support from professionals that they know and trust. So I think the team that's supporting the young adult through to their death has got to be available to them day and night, and weekends, and have access obviously to the appropriate medication and the appropriate skill and expertise to enable them to be in the environment that they want to be. There's nothing worse for a young adult to choose to decide that yes, they ought to die at home with their family, and then to know that in the middle of the night or at weekends they can't actually receive the appropriate care that they deserve.
> (Sarah)

However, Sarah also told me that currently many of these young adults have portacaths, but as district nurses tend to have less expertise with portacaths than with Hickman lines there is often an issue about who is able to care for a patient in the community who has a portacath. However, as Sheila said, even Hickman lines may be unfamiliar to some community-based staff more used to syringe drivers:

> So, for some of our young people, even below the age of sort of 16, Macmillan nurses ... have been involved if they have a cancer diagnosis. Other areas won't get involved until they've gone over 18. Sometimes it's what kind of equipment you need to use, so if they had a Hickman line some of the services won't get involved, because they're very used to using syringe drivers. And so, again, that can impact on who will or will not get involved.
> (Sheila)

The implication here is that the option for services able and willing to support a home death can be dependent on region/location, the combination of services available locally and familiarity with technologies used at the end of life. The age of the young person may mean they fall between children's and adult services, an issue addressed in further detail later in this chapter.

Planning for end of life

Thus far the focus has been on palliative and supportive care in the home rather than specifically 'end of life' care. The literature suggests that planning for the end of life should take place well in advance of the time when the need to access such care may become suddenly urgent. Although this would appear to be good advice, such planning may reflect an ideal set of circumstances that assumes young people and their families will be sure in advance of what they wish for at the end of life and willing to engage with the prospect of death. A family's situation may change, they may plan for a home death that becomes difficult to manage, or they may realise that having decided against a home death, when the time comes it is in fact what they want. The following case study of Tania and her son Dan, who died at home, demonstrates that even for those families who do not plan a home death, the boundary between palliative and end of life care, and the ability to know in advance what will be felt appropriate at the end of life, can be unpredictable.

Case study: Tania and Dan (16) – an unplanned home death

We had meetings regarding his end of life plan and his care, we always planned to have Dan at [the hospice] when he died. We didn't in the end – he stayed here with us, which was against everything we had arranged, really. It just worked out that way, really – he was getting poorlier and poorlier ... we wanted him at home and it just felt right for us. I felt like I put [the hospice] under a lot of pressure by deciding to have him at home. They have said not, they said as a family they understood, with us especially, our desire to be together and be where we felt it was right for us, you know ...? At that point, I think 2 months before he died, we had managed to get his end-of-life plan in place. I don't think the hospital expected it to be quite as quick as it was - whereas [the hospice], they tried to prepare us a lot better. In fact [they] tried to prepare us for about 6 months before that eventuality, if I am honest. The hospital, our consultant, just had different views about ventilators and things that we didn't agree with. It all got a bit rocky at one point when what we wanted and what he felt was beneficial for Dan, it didn't agree. Then Dan started to deteriorate quite a lot, and then he [the consultant] came around to our way of thinking. [The] chest specialist, with his input it really swung the thing round, because he really respected our decision and thought it was the right decision ... I think they had a big multi-agency meeting at the hospital – I think that was in April – and then Dan died at the end of July. I knew he was going for 2.5 months before he died. There was no way his body was going to keep on taking that kind of punishment ... I was scared to have that responsibility on my shoulders, especially with his medication. The weekend he died was the only weekend that the [hospice staff] couldn't be with us ... one was at a wedding I think, and one was somewhere else for the weekend. It was the only weekend that we would have been on our own and couldn't phone anyone. Bearing in mind the home service wasn't up and running properly then, it wasn't as if they had an obligation, but we were scared of moving him in the ambulance ... he could have died in the ambulance ... Plus my husband just so wanted him at home ... In the end a doctor came from the hospice – although I think he might have just been on cover or something. It turned out he only lived about seven or eight doors away. We didn't know he was on the estate, just through here ... he was a lovely man but obviously we didn't have the familiarity ... Luckily my friend is ... a very experienced nurse – and came and gave us a lot of support that weekend. We had big issues over the morphine because I was scared of giving it to him. In the end, when he was in so much pain, I decided to give it to him on the Saturday and it didn't work. I was ringing [the hospice] and saying, 'It has not even stopped him crying out ...' And we ended up having to give him three doses over a space of about 3 or 4 hours ... That was when the syringe driver had to be set up, that afternoon. I think they did as much as they could do, as much as they could do in the circumstances. The fact that we had made it difficult for them in some respects ... I know they say we didn't, but the fact that we changed the goalposts and wanted him at home – I think they were wonderful, really – they did what they could for us. At that point as well, we didn't know whether he was going to pull through. There was still hope, the doctor said he had seen people worse than him pull through, but has seen people better than him die. We just didn't know how it was going to go, but he went the very next day and that was it.

(Tania)

It may be the case that the prospect of a home death for a child or young adult with a long-term life-limiting condition can appear, in principle, difficult to support, but that in the event the 'end of life' care is not significantly different from the care they have received in the home throughout their lives. Problems may arise if services are unavailable but as Tania's account shows, with goodwill this can be overcome if service providers coordinate with one another. In direct contrast, Anne said that a number of the young people she had cared for in the community, who had elected to die at home, in the end died in the hospice because they had been admitted for pain and symptom control and had never been well enough to leave. The problem of delivering effective rapid pain control in the home setting was explained by Anne as follows:

The GP has to write a prescription, it takes you know a day to get the drugs sorted out, so really you're looking you know 2 or 3 days of getting drugs, trying them out, see if they work, and if they don't work. So it's a time factor. If we could give them something, see how it works and then ... [if necessary] try something else, that would be fine; but we can't do that in the community – with whatever resources we're not able to do that. So

really it is about them being in an environment where drugs are on-hand and we can … control that pain.
(Anne)

So it is clear that although it may be good practice to plan for the end of life, in the event, circumstances may result in an unexpected death either at home or in a hospital or hospice. When an unplanned outcome occurs, particularly if the death does not occur at home, it is vital the families are reassured that they have in no way failed or let down their child.

Home-based care for teenagers and young adults with cancer

Although the children with complex and life-limiting conditions may have had an extended period of home-based palliative care, the logical extension of which may be end of life care, for TYAs with cancer the situation may be very different. The prospect of the end of life with cancer may hold fears about the kind of symptoms that have to be managed, the level of pain that may need to be controlled and the need for expertise in the use of technical interventions such as portacaths. Despite such concerns, many of the families who participated in the research, and their sons and daughters, were committed to achieving a home death.

The importance of a home death was emphasised by Hugh's parents, Jonno and Rosie. Rosie told me the following story about the events surrounding her son Hugh's death:

Hugh had wanted a party and we said, 'Yes fine, okay, what do you want?'. He said, 'I want a Guy Fawkes party: lots of fireworks', and he'd been planning this for a couple of months probably. And all of his peer group were off to university, so we got everybody invited before they went, and they were all planning to come. And then he dropped into a coma about 3 days before. And well, there were great discussions amongst all of us about whether it should go on or whether it shouldn't go on. And … we talked to the doctors and we talked to everybody, and they all said, 'Well as long as it's not going to upset him then much better it happens'. And in the end he had half of his care team, half of his doctors, all his friends, and they all went up and said, you know, 'Good luck, mate', and held his hand. They were so brave, I cannot … just can't say how brave they were. And one little girl said, 'Cheerio Hugh, I'll see you tomorrow. I'll come in and see you tomorrow'. … and I said to her when she came out, 'You must go up and you must say that actually … when you come in tomorrow you must tell him that you're going back to university and won't be back 'til Christmas', and she did that the following day. And she went out and she had a little cry and 5 minutes later he took a last breath … And he really wanted that party. The fact that we could have it home was wonderful.

(Rosie)

Hugh's parents attributed the 'good death' they achieved for their son to the excellent relationship between local hospital services and the outreach nurses who supported him in their home. Jonno said he believed that if Hugh's primary treatment centre (PTC) had been at their regional hospital, a 2-hour drive away from their home, they could never have achieved the collaboration and cooperation on which the shared care between the local hospital and community care was based (this issue of shared care is further explored in Chapter 4). However, Hugh's death did not occur as and when they had expected, and their decision to continue with the party despite the decline in Hugh's condition shows a commitment to respecting what his parents believed he would have wanted – a party surrounded by his friends and the people who mattered to him – after all what harm could it do? This last question is reminiscent of Sue Grant's (2005) decision about her son Alexander's end of life care at home. Despite the healthcare professionals' warnings against a home death, she was determined to support Alexander's death at home. It was not without difficulties but enabled Alexander and his family to take control of the end of his life and do the things that were important to them while ignoring the things that intruded. They decided on their priorities in the same way as Jonno and Rosie, as Sue describes:

> Because I could not make him well again I felt helpless. But being able to support him in his wish to die in the familiarity of his own home with his family around him was a great consolation ... Our daily routine relaxed. He didn't want the dressing on his thin arm changed today? Fine. Let's do it tomorrow. Or not at all. It didn't matter anymore ... Instead we had lots of time to exchange memories, to be close together, undisturbed by the noise and inevitable hectic environment of a hospital ward ... Both of us – mother and father – camped on the living-room floor that final night. His brother and sister waited upstairs. So when the end came, we could hardly have asked for a more beautiful one. We were all with him and could let him go peacefully, gently and with great dignity. Am I glad that I did it. (Sue Grant 2005: 13)

The importance of an age-appropriate approach

The following two stories of Billie and Ellen's deaths raise issues about home deaths that have both similarities and differences, but both show how important relationships with care providers are in making the decision that a home death is possible. They also show that, even outside the paediatric or adult settings of inpatient care, an age-appropriate approach is of fundamental importance.

Billie's story

Billie, at 14, was younger than many young people who chose a home death, but she knew she was going to die and was no less clear in her strong wish to die at home. Unlike Jonno and Rosie's account, in which shared care was successful, Billie's mother Beckie told me the following about her daughter's home death in which shared care with the local hospital broke down:

> She just wanted to go home ... she wanted to go home, so that's what we did. We had very good community nursing, because we'd been having that all the way through her illness anyway, so we knew them really well. So that was lucky for us, because I know that people who, once they've left the hospital, they had to get to know a whole new load of people that they'd never met before in their lives ... Her dad went to stay with her for a few days [in hospital] and I came home to get the house ready for her. And while I was at home I phoned the local hospice, because we're very lucky where we are, we've got two hospices ... I phoned them and they just told me, 'It's not a problem if you need to come in'. Because I knew she didn't want to go to hospital, and there's no way on God's earth I was going to take her to [the district general hospital, DGH], not in a million years I was going to take her to shared-care hospital. She was so desperate to go home she started crying. I never really thought, 'Oh my God she's crying because she's going to die ...', and she was going, 'I can go home. I can go', and she was happy. She was crying because she was happy because she could go home, can you believe it ... ? I bought everything pink, and fluffy, and sparkly available in East London. So I decorated all down the stairs like a big boudoir.
>
> (Beckie)

Despite the relationship with the DGH having broken down (see Chapter 4), Beckie had the assurance that hospice care would be available if necessary. This was an essential backup for her peace of mind as Beckie said that no one would tell her what to expect when Billie died as *'they won't talk about it'*, and she was afraid Billie's pain or other symptoms would be traumatic and out of control. But Billie's home death was achieved in the reassuring home setting so important to her, with the support of the community nursing service who Beckie told me had access to equipment unavailable at the local hospital, such as a self-regulated morphine pump. The ongoing importance of a home death for Billie and her ability to provide it helped to sustain Beckie in her bereavement, and she emphasises its significance as follows:

> I think being able to do what Billie wanted was the most important thing in the whole world, and that's enabled me to sleep at night. And I can't imagine what it would be like not to have that. That must be ... I really couldn't ... it's horrific to me, the idea that she could have ended her life in an A & E cubicle, which some ... you know must happen, with people not knowing her, and not understanding her, and not knowing me and asking me to get out the way, you know. But she didn't; she died on the sofa in our living room, with me and my husband, and ... you know and that ... I can't ... if our kids have to die then surely [they] deserve to do it the way [they] need to do it. I can't imagine anybody deserving it more really.
>
> (Beckie)

Ellen's story

Ann's daughter Ellen at 23 was also determined to die at home – the account of her distressing visit to an adult hospice is documented in Chapter 3. Indeed it seems for both Billie and Ellen, the distress caused by their experiences in a hospital (Billie) and hospice (Ellen) meant that the desire to be cared for at home was particularly strong. Although 14-year-old Billie's death was in a 'pink and fluffy and sparkly' setting, the way Ellen managed her death at home could also be interpreted as 'age-related'. Her mother, Ann, told me:

> When she left the hospital and we drove home she decided that she was going to watch *Friends*. And she watched *Friends* continuously from when we got home to when she died – or virtually when she died [about a month] ... day and night ... to start with it wasn't continuous, because ... if we wanted to watch something else we did all watch things together; we watched films with her. And she liked going out in the car so I used to take her out in the car and we'd just drive. She'd just tell me where to drive and we'd do that. But ... as she became more poorly, she wanted to watch it later and into the night, and she slept with me but she wanted to sleep downstairs and watch the television. So I used to sleep downstairs with her ... it was just something that she wanted to do ... it had to be her way ... Ellen was very much in control. [Friends] did visit – more so when we first got home rather than latterly ... it was difficult for her brother and sister, but ... they did go and sit with her and, you know ... and probably this is why she did it [watch television], it did make it easier for everyone, because we could ... go and sit with her but we didn't have to talk about anything. You know, we could just be with her and ... we'd talk about what was happening on the television at that time or ... and that really carried on ... until a couple of days before she died.
>
> (Ann)

Ann told me how supportive her GP had been, Ellen had allowed him to carry her upstairs via a spiral staircase a few hours before she died even though she would not let her father do this. Ann said this GP was *'very, very good in the last few weeks'*. Here, Ann describes how Ellen's pain relief was managed at home:

> There were some occasions when her pain went up in the night and then in the morning I just had this Post-It saying you know, tell Sarah [her community-based nurse] I need some more morphine ... She had a lot of pain.
>
> (Ann)

Sarah, who was also present at my interview with Ann, said about the management of Ellen's pain:

> Her symptom control was quite difficult actually because she had horrendous vomiting ... and she had an horrendous obstruction ... There were a few times when it was on the edge I think, but ... we were fortunate with the consultant at [the PTC], we used a lot of drugs outside of licensing, which I think helped. And really, up until a few days before Ellen died, she was very much in control. Whatever you did to Ellen she always wanted to know exactly what you were doing and why you were doing it. But probably 3, 4 days before she died I said to her what I was doing and she said, 'I don't want to know anymore, just get on with it, just do it', and that was quite significant. That was a real change. She didn't want any more explaining. I think she'd had ... enough. It was just a case of control it, do it, get on with it, don't tell me anymore. But I think we did control symptoms ... you had good support really – the out of hours service, the district nurses.
>
> (Sarah)

Ann then told me the hospice at home service did not offer 24-hour support so for the rest of the time that the district nurses cared for Ellen, coming in the morning to change her syringe driver. Although both Ann and Sarah felt that the pain control and home-based support had been well managed and that Ellen's death at home had been well supported, it seems that the attitude of some of the community nurses was perceived by Ellen as patronising, and when this was the case she did not want them to attend to her any more. Sarah mentioned the following exchange, which she felt had been inappropriately handled by a district nurse. What Ellen needed at that time was planning for the things she could still do rather than for death:

> The very first visit we did to Ellen was a joint visit. Because of her age we had a joint visit with an adult CNS (community nursing service) who sat there and, on the very first visit, asked Ellen how much she understood about her prognosis and that she would die from her illness. And I was sat opposite the table and that's not how I'd do a visit ... and Ellen, you could see, was biting back the tears – it was awful. And this nurse left before me and she [Ellen] said, 'I don't ever want her to come back', and that was it, she'd closed the door ... she didn't want, on a first visit, to talk about that. We talked about how we could get a car on the mobility.
>
> (Sarah)

It may be that in this instance, in an attempt to treat Ellen as an adult – which she clearly was at 23 – the nurse had misunderstood Ellen's need to live her life as fully as possible in the relatively short time she had left. A young adult facing death in her early 20s requires a different approach from that which might be offered to an older adult, thus an age-appropriate approach is important if the relationship between the young person and their health care providers is to offer them the best experience, and indeed not result in the young person refusing treatment from a professional who gets it wrong.

Ellen's refusal to allow the nurse to return demonstrates the importance of an age-appropriate approach in this age group. Conversely, Joan reported that her son Stuart, who was nearly 18, was inappropriately treated like a child. Although Stuart was not in the end able to die at home, which would have been his preference; this was his mother's account of his experience of home care:

> You know he just didn't like the invasion of home, of nurses coming twice a week to do his bloods. He found it a pain. And unfortunately, because they are community nurses they treat ... and they used to see some little children – they treated him as if he was about six.
> (Joan)

A home death must be supported by excellent community-based services and it was the absence of having assured home care in place that meant Joan was prevented from taking her son Stuart home to die. This was despite the fact that the hospital was in the throes of a crisis and wished to discharge him:

> They had a major thing come in – I think there'd been an attack or something – so they wanted him out of there, because there was police and all sorts. And they said actually ... we can't let you go home. And I said, 'Well please, I just want to take him home ... I just want to take him home'. And they said, 'You can't because you haven't got the backup from a Macmillan nurse, and we can't get hold of anybody'.
> (Joan)

Joan told me she would have been able to take Stuart home had the Macmillan nurse not been on holiday, so Joan's inability to provide a home death for Stuart appears to have rested on the unfortunate temporary absence of a Macmillan nurse.

Ian's story

Although in US terminology Ian's death was a 'hospice death', I have included it in this chapter as hospice deaths in America take place in the home supported by community-based care. Ian died at 23 from oesophageal cancer at home in the USA, against medical advice. His doctor said to his mother Laura: 'Are you really sure that you want to do this?' He was, Laura told me, 'concerned for us personally, as to how we were gonna manage Ian ... '. Ian had insisted – against advice - on being discharged from the hospital where his parents hoped he would remain for his end of life care (see Chapter 5). His mother had not wanted hospice services to be involved in his end of life care at home, but it was the condition upon which his discharge took place. The following extract from my interview with Laura and her husband Arthur gives an account of the challenges the family faced:

Laura

I fought for every single thing I could get for him, and when they decided on hospice I was dead set against hospice. I was gonna take him home and take care of him by myself, because I already knew – and I knew in the last couple of weeks that this was gonna come down to this ... I didn't want those people in my house 'cos I know what they're about, and they ... I asked for somebody that had experience, people that had experience with young adults and they ... they flat-out lied through their teeth to us, just to get us to take the hospice care on, and I finally did. I refused to sign any papers, I said, 'He's old enough to sign his own papers. I'm not signing any, you know, "Do not resuscitates"; I'm not signing anything ...'.

Hospice in, at least in Massachusetts, is, you know, it's a privately-run business organisations that provide service ... Sort of like if you wanted to get the house cleaned you'd hire somebody and they'd come in with, you know, the staff and they'd do it, and that's what hospice care is, in Boston in Massachusetts, and probably in the United States – I don't think there's any Government-run – there might be I don't know, but in my experiences both professionally and personally, hospice is a travesty, it's a farce ... But they were contracted to the hospital. We didn't have any other choice, and I said on a number of occasions, 'I'll take him home without you. I don't need your help. I can get ... a hospital bed; I can get the equipment that I need', and they right-out told me that I couldn't take him home unless I signed on to hospice, or he signed on to hospice.

Ian went through the hospice process, and we didn't have a great experience with hospice ... my personal feeling about hospice is that it's a money-making organisation that provides whatever care it has to ... There is some emotional support, but, the kinds of things that they were pushing at us, like, 'Oh, you know, we're gonna make this a great death experience for him'. It's like, 'You don't understand ... he doesn't plan on dying'.

I've got training in caring for people ... I have a background in occupational therapy. I don't do that anymore, but I have a background in it and I've cared for people most of my life, so I don't have a problem with that. I think he got to a point where he was very comfortable with the dressing of ... a slight wound on his tailbone, and he didn't have a problem ... with letting me deal with that, 'cos I know he knew that I was being professional ... so it wasn't embarrassing for him ... I don't think it was ever about embarrassment, I think it was about control ... and being able to [do] those functions himself without anybody helping him.

Arthur

The problem with home hospice is you in effect become the care giver: they give you the ... medical equipment and the medications but you'll be, in effect, become the nurse, and it doesn't give you the opportunity to be the grieving parent, the grieving son, or to just be ... the family member. You in effect have to change roles and take out emotion. As far as the storybook endings with ... his family ... around him when he was dying ... me and my wife were here when he died, and it's not a pleasant thing ... it's not a storybook ending ... the hospice said they'd have medication for us: the first day it wasn't there, the second day they were here ... they asked if it was okay if they didn't come every single day.

Laura

They promised us ... his doctor told us he needed to have an IV to go home ... Hospice said, 'Oh, not a problem. We can get him an IV'. ... He came home, they told us, 'Oh, well, we can't do an IV', ... And we were, like, 'What?'... with this type of cancer, he can't swallow... they agreed to get ... things for us, and then every single thing we asked for they found a way to excuse themselves from.

With regards to the IV pole, they said they'd just do it, and I think the problem was, even though I think they had registered nurses who could administer IVs, the home care people don't have that level of expertise to do an IV, I think [that] was the problem ... I could have done it myself ... he had a port ... in his chest ... and once that [was] open ... any one of us could have put in atropine through that ... and made that death a lot less horrific than it was, because he struggled, at the very end ... if we had been able to push that medication ... we saw him in the hospital nearly asphyxiate, and that was when my husband said, 'I don't want to see my son die like that'. And that's exactly how our son died ... exactly the way he didn't want to ... And that's what the doctor had tried to prevent - he tried to protect us from that but, you know, we wanted to take Ian home because that's what Ian said he wanted ...

Ian's mother - against her better judgment - agreed to allow hospice services to support his home death. However, as she suspected, the service was unreliable and did not take into account that this would be the death of a young man who had no intention of dying. Paradoxically, the very thing she feared at the end of his life was what transpired. Thus it seems that in the USA, despite such community-based services being privatised and paid for, their quality, expertise and ability to support the technologies used routinely at the end of life, may be in question.

The inconsistency of community-based provision

It became apparent from the data collected in the UK that a minority of participants had experienced difficulties in obtaining community-based services and that some young people fell through the gap between paediatric and adult services. Val's story about her son Martin's home death raises troubling issues relating to home-based care for 16–18-year olds in the UK and is presented as a case study.

Case study: Martin's story

Martin was discharged from the PTC after treatment options had failed; his prognosis suggested he had a very short time to live, and he and his family wanted that time to be spent at home and for him to be able to die there with appropriate support. This is his mother's account of the period leading up to and after his discharge from a London teaching hospital:

> They said they will be able to give you information about the services that are going to be available to take care of you from now on in your own community. So I went to see somebody, and this nurse explained that very recently the method of funding had been changed. So it had been that [the] Hospital, and the children's ward, and TCT (Teenage Cancer Trust), along with [another] hospital had had a pot of funding and anyone within those hospitals – any of the children or young people in those hospitals – if they were going to die at home, there was a pot of money that those hospitals could allocate to go with them to whatever services they needed. And she said that's been changed now, so that we still have that pot of money but we can only spend it on people who live in two London boroughs. And so we can't spend it on Martin because he lives outside of London. So she said this is a very new change and this is ... she said this is I think the first time – certainly the first time they'd dealt with our area. And she said, so I now have to find out what's available. So it wasn't a case of, 'Come and let me tell you what's available'. It's, 'I'm going to have to find out what's available'. And ... she wasn't skilled at doing it; she didn't know what she was going to be doing.
>
> So that was bad enough, right. So we went home. I think I started making sure that I was ringing regularly to say, 'Well, where have you got [to], what's happening?'. And then of course I discovered what she hadn't told me at that point; she probably didn't really dare to tell me in front of Martin, or didn't want to tell us. She ... didn't want to tell us. But in a conversation with her it suddenly became clear that if there is any money locally to spend on his care, children's services pay for the care of children up to the age of 16. This includes children's hospices and ... whatever – up to the age of 16. Adult services provide for people from the age of 18 – you're not allowed to die aged 17. And if you do you don't exist, and if you do there's no provision for you whatsoever.

And I was absolutely horrified. It was the most awful feeling. I knew that Martin was in pain; I knew he couldn't breathe; I knew ... he wasn't on oxygen by then. I knew that he had breathing problems, I knew the cancer was in his bones and in his lungs. So he wasn't going to be able to breathe, and I believe the cancer ... a lot of people say cancer in the bones is about as painful as cancer can get. This was going to happen to my child. There was no way he was going to go into hospital. He didn't want to be in hospital. And yet how were we going to get any provision? So I spent my time phoning everybody that I could, saying, 'What's going to happen? Do something! Everybody do something!'. What I really wanted to do was ring the people who'd made that funding decision and scream at them and say, 'Come and sit with my child while he dies and see how you feel'.

(Val)

In the event, there was home-based support for Martin that enabled him to die at home, but it was stitched together from a variety of sources all of whom pulled together to bridge the gap in services. This is Val's account of how support was coordinated unofficially:

Because there were no official services for him, everybody who heard about his situation eventually said we want to help. ... our GP obviously was involved, but our GP was on holiday so another GP from the practice came. We had the palliative care consultant from Marie Curie Hospice, which is 10 minutes away. She was able to come to our house ... but he couldn't go there because of his age. For a couple of hours we had a couple of the nurses from the Marie Curie Hospice ... We had two people from the children's hospice ... which is a good hour's journey away. Now if Martin had decided I don't want to be here [at home] I do want to be in a hospice that would be where he would have to go – another hour's journey by ambulance.

(Val)

It seems that Martin's home death was facilitated by the compassion and goodwill of local care providers who were prevailed upon by a knowledge-able and articulate parent who, in her own words, had to undergo the additional stress of 'phoning everybody that I could, saying, 'What's going to happen? Do something! Everybody do something!'. This reported lack of provision for a young person aged between 16 and 18 clearly raises many concerns. As a result of Val's account, I attempted to discover how widespread the gap in the provision of home-based care for 16-18-year-olds is.

I began by interviewing Gill, the Clinical Services Co-ordinator for Long Term Conditions in community nursing in a city in the North West of England. She was somewhat surprised by my question about the lack of services for 16–18-years-olds and said the following:

> We see anybody who's got a nursing need and we do all the end of life care in the community ... I can only speak for my locality, but we would nurse an individual, a palliative care person, however old they were, be they, you know, five, seven, 16, 18, 19, up to being 110. They would get the same service ... So, if they meet our criteria, i.e. they are housebound and they have a nursing need, then we'll see them ... The district nursing service ... give quite a comprehensive service in so far as we are 24 hours a day, 7 days a week. And patients can ring at any time, day or night, if they have an issue or they have a concern. We work collaboratively with the acute trust and the hospice, and the hospice have an outreach service as well. So people can get core district nursing service and it can be topped up, for want of a better word, with outreach, with Marie Curie ... [and] Macmillan operate here as well ... they're actually funded jointly by [the] PCT [primary care trust], and the hospice put some money in as well. But I assign money to them so it means that, you know, at the professional meetings we have district nurses, community matrons, all the specialist nurses including the Macmillan team. So they see themselves as being part of the same workforce and that is really helpful.
> (Gill)

Although it was clear that in this North West city home-based care services were available to support this age group, Gill acknowledged that caring for young people of this age at the end of their lives raised some issues for the staff. She told me about the case of a young man whose peaceful home death had been supported by a team who had been profoundly affected by it: 'The clinical supervision afterwards was quite emotional, because I think ... that the team perhaps got more closely involved with the care of that young man and his family, because of his youth' (Gill). She added that caring for a dying young adult was so unusual and so 'against nature' that the team had gone 'the extra mile'.

Having established that in this locality there appeared to be no gap in provision – indeed it could be argued that provision for the age group was even more carefully delivered – it seemed there was nevertheless a nationwide inconsistency. I continued to ask a wide variety of health professionals I met at conferences, or who were formally interviewed research participants, what the provision in their region was like. The results showed patchiness across the country. For example, nurses at one age-specific unit in a large city in the North of England told me that it was not until they looked at the postcode of the patient they planned to discharge with a care package for end of life support in the community that they knew if care would be available; this was verified by the paediatric consultant from this locality whom I consulted on a separate occasion.

Although use of home-based services was, of course, more usual for the children with complex and life-limiting conditions, most of whom at the age of 16 would continue to receive the services they had had throughout their life, a professional from a different region in the UK told me that in her area there would be home-based care for the 16-18-year-old with cancer but not for a young person with chronic life-limiting illness. Thus, it seems that this age group can fall into a gap between services regardless of their illness depending on where they live, and that in some locations there will be services for cancer patients but not others, whereas the reverse can be true in other geographical areas.

Concern about the patchiness of community-based care was also expressed in some of the responses to the service evaluation questionnaires I distributed to every TCT unit in the UK in 2009. The extracts from the questionnaires, below, show the range of responses reflecting variation in local provision:

'There are examples of very good care and examples of not so good care.'

'For 16-18 years our outreach paediatric team will still monitor and take care of patients at home. We are in the process of employing a TYA CNS nurse to look after patient end of life needs from those aged 16-25 years, which will include some home care and organisation of home care at end of life.'

'Adult community palliative care services are well established in our region and provide an excellent service, which we hope would extend to the group of 16-18-year-olds when the need arises.'

'Home-based support is mixed but on the whole can be arranged if necessary with good rapid discharge team and system if needed.'

'Depends on where they live'

'Varies from area to area'

'I think that the 16-18-year-olds are a particularly tricky group, as with some services there may be disagreement as to which service the patient falls into.'

From the additional service evaluation carried out by Grinyer and Barbarachild (2011) the following responses echoed those above:

Home, hospital, hospice if appropriate – but not 16-18-yr-olds.

There's still a debate about 17-year-olds. They are often outside children's services but not old enough for adult services. 17-year-olds fall out of both camps.

Grinyer and Barbarachild (2011: 11)

In addition to the gap for 16–18-year-olds being cared for at home, Rosemarie (from an adult hospice in the South East of the UK) indicated that there could also be a gap in skills for home-based care for the over 18 s:

> The community services haven't … caught up with the younger people coming through, because we've not been used to it. We've either had young children with cancer who've had treatment and survived or have died, or we've had adults … What we do find is, from 18+ the community nurses don't necessarily have all of the skills that would be needed to enable someone to have their treatment at home, to have their bloods taken at home … the ports [portacaths] that they have, because the adult patients don't have them, so the adult district nurses aren't used to caring for these kind of sort of physical aspects. And because they see very few sort of young adults with malignancies, they don't see enough to keep their skills up, so that's proving to be a problem at the moment. So we're in the position now where you know you hit 18 and the cut-off point, and actually then from having been nursed at home, you know these young people are having to get on the train and go to London to get ports flushed and things like that … [it's] a real trek. It's not an easy journey … and quite often the burden for that falls on parents, friends, because actually hospital transport just to get bloods, it's nonsensical really because if you were able to get it you would be waiting around all day to get back home again. So it's got to be either public transport or reliant on friends and family. So you know the burden isn't just on the patient, it's on their support network as well.
> (Rosemarie)

Rosemarie suggested that rather than services being seamlessly joined to eliminate the gap, it would be better if they overlapped. She said she struggled with the rather dismissive attitude: '"Oh, it's palliative care", so it gets pushed to the palliative care service and not really grasped by the community. We're having a bit of a wrangle at the moment getting the community services to take ownership of this issue'.

Death in a marital home

Thus far the discussion of end of life care and death at home has focused on it taking place in the parental home. However, the young adult age group, particularly young adults with cancer, are of an age and at a life-stage when they may be married or living with a partner. The delicacy of the relationships when a son or daughter is dying in their 'marital' home, rather than living with their family of origin, can be challenging for parents. When and how long to be present, sharing care and support, and who has responsibility for decision making: all these issues can require skilled negotiations at a time when those close to the dying young adult are distressed and anxious.

The case study involving Pat's daughter Sara demonstrates how a good death can be achieved, that both respects the wishes of the young adult and her partner and also acknowledges the needs of the parents and siblings – but it does not gloss over the difficulties. This example from Canada gives a non-UK perspective. Sara was 26 when she died; the account also mentions Sara's father Lee, her sister Jenny and her husband Brad.

Case study: Pat's daughter Sara's death in her marital home

She wanted to die at home with her husband and her cat. And so we arranged for them to be in their condominium, we arranged for a hospice care doctor to come in so that she didn't have to go to get that kind of assistance at the end of her life. And it also prepared us a family that once she did die we would call that doctor and they would come in and make up the certification of her death ... She did not need to be in a medical facility for end of life care, in terms of her physicality of what was happening to her. Slowly everything was just shutting down and we were aware of that because she quit eating, she quit drinking. And it was important for us to understand that was a natural process of when some-one's dying that happens ... The hospice nurses ... came in on a daily basis or on our request. If there was any concern about her medication or if she was in distress, we were able to call people in to help us assist her through her process ... This is in Canada, in British Columbia; I don't [know] ... how that's covered elsewhere.

Just a few days before Sara died; all of a sudden she decided she needed to go back to the hospital. And we called in her doctor, to talk to her about it, because we would be willing to do that. We were trying to just always listen to what Sara needed. It was important that she control that as much as she could, right to the very end. So we didn't deny it, we just questioned why all of a sudden this was happening to her. So this hospice doctor, who was very aware of how to care for people, who knew about this process ... was familiar with what the distress might be for Sara. And all of a sudden Sara got in her mind, for some reason, that if she went to the hospital she would be able to eat again. If she went to the hospital she'd be able to sleep again and be at rest. And the third thing was that her pain would be less. So what the doctor did was, she just was very matter of fact and agreed with Sara that these are concerns and then she proceeded to say that 'if you go to a hospital you realise you'll be ... lights will be on, it'll be loud, you may not be in a private room and so your ability to sleep might not be any better than what we can do for you here, which is just to up your meds if that's what's needed'. The thing about the eating, she said, 'Sara, you know, what would you like to eat, because if there's something we're not providing for you ... we can pro-vide it here at your home'. And then the pain thing was easily managed.

Once Sara had an opportunity to talk about these things, with this person she trusted, she decided that she really didn't want to go to the hospital after all. And that was a great relief to all of us because we felt that we would love for her to be at home so we could be with her. However, as I said, our job was to make sure that we would follow her requests, so had she actually, even after the discussion, chosen to go back to the hospital, where she would have died, because this was just days, if not the day before she died, that we would have done that with her. But again we kept going back, and so did the doctors say, 'You know your request was that you would die at home with Brad your husband and your father and your sister, and your mother and your cat'.

Well, actually I have to clarify that, she wanted just to die with her husband and her cat, but she meant to include us in the fact that we would not be able to be with her and visit with her as easily [in hospital] as we could when we were in their home.

And that seemed to calm Sara down; she just seemed to need to know … that going to the hospital wasn't going to stop her from dying … So it was a last-ditch effort of being connected to what Sara thought might save her life would be, 'I'd better go to the hospital if I don't want to die'. … So your home care team, whoever that involves, it's really important they be involved with the patient before they get to the end of life – because just they might be saying things at the very end that would need to be attended to in a different way than what they'd said 2 or 3 weeks prior.

The one thing through the process of preparing for her to die that was important to her is that sometimes we would – like we'd always do in a family dynamic – we would talk to her about what she was feeling about Brad, and that was mum and sister kind of talk, about your relationship. Then she would talk to Brad about his relationship with our family. And finally it got to the point where she sat us both down, all of us down together one day, and said, 'I can no longer be in the middle of this. I cannot be your mediator. You have to talk to each other'. So we did. We had to. It wasn't always easy but we found a way … I feel that Brad feels that we were as much of a support as we could be. And as we talk now, in 10 years retrospect, we're more forgiving of each other, of the times that we didn't always agree because we had our own agenda and our own connections with Sara. And I think that intellectually we understood that, but emotionally … we weren't always in sync. But, in retrospect, I think yes, we all feel that if you can say it was a good death, that Sara's was a good death. And we were part of that. And she invited us in, in the way that she could. That was an incredible gift.

She did allow us to be there up until … the night before she died; it was a very funny situation. They had a little courtyard outside their condo and … we'd go out and then we came back and we'd always come back and say goodnight. And that was the night we came back and Brad said,

'She's gone to bed, she doesn't want to say goodnight'. And then we went out and we were talking in the courtyard and she yelled out through the courtyard doors, and she said, 'Have they left yet?', and we just broke up laughing because that was just so typical of Sara. But really I do believe ... she was literally waiting for us to leave before she could die. That's my interpretation of that. I believe that very strongly. And she wanted us to respect that ... I remember saying to Lee on the way home that night ... 'If Sara dies tonight, Jenny's going to be pretty upset', because she was angry that Brad wouldn't let her in. And she did die. We got a call the next morning, at 7:30, to say that she'd passed on and that we were to go down. And I remember asking Jenny, just recently, whether she actually felt that way when he had said that, and she said 'no' ... she felt that Sara also had made her wishes clear – die alone with my husband and my cat and that was what she did.

You know this is the difference about being a mother of a young adult with cancer, whose primary care-giver was her husband. And they'd only been married a year and a bit. They'd lived together but when she got cancer – 10 October 1997, that's when she was diagnosed – and she reclaimed that day, the following 10 October 1998, to be married so she could make that day a joyous day. She died in the summer of 2000 – July 2000. So it wasn't very long they were actually married. However I'd already had to accept the fact that that was her primary carer.

So when she died we knew we were going to bathe her and we were going to dress her in her wedding dress. And the funny thing about it was that the rigor mortis set in, which I think we all knew because we'd seen enough movies about that, but to dress her when she's stiff – we didn't know that if we had waited a few hours that she might have relaxed. So there was a bit of humour about it all.

The other thing, which was a bit of a startling thing for us, and had we been prepared for it ahead of time it would have been helpful ... is that when we turned her to bathe her on the back side of her body, I didn't know that when people died the contents of their stomach somehow gurgle up and will come out of the mouth and it's very putrid smelling. Now whether that was directly from her medications and her cancer, or whether that's a normal thing, I don't know. I never asked anyone since then. But fortunately ... her father was there, and he had a towel so he sort of covered it up ... Well it was just that we weren't prepared ...

And the other thing was is that her colour ... yes she was very pale but she was absolutely, extremely beautiful and people often talk about how peaceful their loved one looked. Well I didn't think Sara looked peaceful because her face was so thin by this time and sunken. I would not have said that she looked peaceful, but her body looked very beautiful in her dress and her feet became like little china doll, ivory feet. And it was interesting because it was her feet that she always asked us to hold in her process of dying. That was the last way we could ground her to this earth consciousness. And it was her feet that were the most beautiful at the end.

As a mother, when the young adult [is] dying ... it was hard for me to give up that primary care-giver relationship to Brad ... Well there were times when Jenny and I both felt it – Jenny primarily because she felt she had known her sister for 26 years, and the relationship with Brad and Sara was still quite new, and there was even the question of you know, if they stayed together – like would they stay together or did he stay with her because she has cancer. They were in love, they loved one another deeply, and he was an amazing supporter of her, so in that regard it was easier to let go of the control of wanting to be the primary care-giver, because Brad was like a trained nurse, even though he was an actor like Sara. He was fantastic. And no one could fault him. The hard role he had was being the person that stood at the bedroom door and said, after Sara had gone to bed, 'She doesn't want to say goodnight to you tonight. She's ready for bed'. ... I think Jenny primarily felt sort of angry at Brad ... once in a while, just 'How can you dictate how to say goodnight to my sister?' But he was only telling us what Sara said and/or translating what he thought Sara said. And we had to totally trust him when he made those kind of calls.

(Pat)

I use this detailed account because it raises many issues about the relation-ship between the family of origin and the marital family. Although Sara's death took place in the home she shared with her husband, it is clear that Pat's use of the term 'we' in the first paragraph means that she and Sara's father and sister were very involved in the arrangements. Yet repeatedly in the account, despite their good relationship, Pat says how difficult it was to accept that Sara's husband Brad was the primary care-giver and 'controlled' access to Sara. This case study also has much to tell us about all home deaths: the importance of professionals knowing what the dying person's wishes are so that if they panic, as Sara did, they are not taken to hospital thus relin-quishing their true wish to die at home; that if the family want to lay out the body they need some practical knowledge of how and when rigor mortis sets in and when they might expect it to pass, and that they will need to manage the secretion of bodily fluids.

Although Pat's account acknowledges the challenges, it is predominantly positive in that goodwill was maintained, she and her family still have a good relationship with Brad, and Sara achieved her wish to die at home with her husband and her cat. Yet we have to remember that Pat was the mother of a daughter who was dying – might the dynamics have been different if she had been the mother of a son? The old adage, 'A son is a son till he takes him a wife, a daughter is a daughter all of her life' (author unknown), may be stereo-typical in its depiction of family relationships, but might also reflect the reality of many mothers' relationships with their married sons. This dynamic is likely to be exacerbated in a home death where the daughter-in-law becomes the gatekeeper, rather than the professionals in a hospice or hospital setting.

Ryan and Bianca's story

In a variation of that scenario, the young married couple Bianca and Ryan, had no option but to support Ryan's end of life care in his mother's home. In Bianca's account of her husband Ryan's death it is evident that her relatively recent status as his wife contributed to a power struggle between her and his mother. Bianca married her long-term boyfriend Ryan only 6 weeks before his death and, as a couple, they were both very resistant to him being cared for in either a hospice or a hospital ward or (see Chapters 3 and 4), so a home death was the only acceptable option to them. Ryan, a recent graduate, and Bianca, an undergraduate, could not afford their own accommodation, so Ryan returned to his mother's house to be cared for, where he had a morphine pump and a respite nurse who came to stay overnight. However, in her interview Bianca did not focus primarily on his medical care, but on the difficulties in managing 'control' of her and his mother's competing relationship with Ryan.

Case study: Ryan and Bianca in Ryan's mother's home

He lived with his dad ... and when he became poorly he had to go and move back in with his mum because his dad worked and his mum was unemployed ... and I was at university, so there was more scope for her to take care of him at home ... She'd been his main carer when he was ill the first time and ... there was more space at his mum's house ... It worked because ... where she lived, it was the doctors and the primary care trust that had cared for him the first time round, so they knew, they had his records, you know, that everything was there, people knew them, the family was known and so ... for him to have been anywhere else, like out of the borough or whatever [would] have been difficult. It was just that was the best place ... and unfortunately it was, it was ... horrible ... but it was, you know, the best, the best option ... It was just ... it was strained because he didn't agree with a lot of the things that she [his mother] did, like she smoked, she was unemployed, she didn't want to get a job ... His mind worked in a very different way and he had very different values from his mum ... so I think it was, that was what made the relationship strained because he didn't always agree with her and her behaviour ...

His mum and I fell out and we don't particularly speak any more. His parents were separated [but] his dad – I think the whole way through the entire cancer experience, when I was involved – always looked at us as 'Bianca and Ryan', and always made provisions for us as 'Bianca and Ryan' ... Whenever we were with his dad's side of the family, I was always factored into any ... trip, appointment at the hospital. I would always stay with Ryan overnight, so his dad was very accepting of my role, and I think he knew how much Ryan wanted me there and how much I meant to Ryan, and so when Ryan was dying and after his death, he was always just, like, 'It's up to Bianca', and that really didn't go down well with his mum ... because in those last stages [in hospital] she never really came to visit him ... and she never really attended any of the appointments ... it was always his dad that took us ... until, like, the final sort of stages, and then suddenly she wanted to be really involved and she wanted to look after her child ... and it became, like, I felt she became very competitive towards the end about who did this for him and who did that, and to the point I was just like ... 'I really don't care, like, I'll back off', you know ... 'If it means that much, you know, that you need to go and give him his drink ...' Then when he died she wanted to be in charge of everything, and his dad was, like, 'Well, you can't anymore, because ... Ryan wasn't a little boy ... he was a grown young man and he made ... choices that mean you're not the first person'. And the fact [was] that Ryan and his mum had a really tempestuous relationship anyway ...

(Bianca)

The lack of choice is summed up by Bianca's phrase 'It was horrible ... but it was the best option'. In addition to the strain between Bianca and Ryan and his mother, Bianca's account reminds us, in the following quote, of Beckie's and Pat's comments about not knowing enough about the physical process of death and its aftermath.

I didn't feel prepared ... like there's a process, like when, you know, as to when someone dies the body shuts down and they become unconscious and they ... their breathing becomes really erratic and I didn't understand any of that process. So when that was happening to him ... there was, there was nurses and whatever that were coming and going to the home, but no one explained to me ... I didn't understand this process. I didn't know this was his body shutting down and it was only in hindsight, when I came back and I questioned people, and I said, 'I don't understand: tell me what happened. Why didn't you tell me this at the time? Why did no-one explain it?' No one ever sat me down and ... spoke to me as an adult ... because people were talking to his parents and his parents were too scared to come and talk to me ... we had a doctor around and they were, like, 'You need to call a Priest'. We're a Catholic family and I was, like, 'No. I don't want a Priest - that means death'.

(Bianca)

That Bianca had not accepted that Ryan would die is discussed in further detail in Chapter 5, but this quote indicates that the professionals spoke with Ryan's parents, rather than to Bianca as his wife. This is clearly age-related and challenged Bianca's centrality and status as Ryan's spouse in a way that might be considered insensitive and inappropriate and unlikely to have happened had they been an older couple.

The implications of supporting a home death

All the examples cited in this chapter thus far have been of cases where a home death was the preference of the young person and/or their family. Although some of the examples have illustrated problems and challenges, none of the participants has indicated that they wished they had opted for an alternative. As we have seen in the summary of the literature, there is an embedded assumption that a home death results in 'the best outcome'. However, such an assumption may place pressure on families to support a death at home about which they feel ambivalent. The age and life-stage of parents of children and young adults may make it appear that they have the physical and emotional resources to support a home death with confidence. However, it is not only the impact on the parents that needs to be considered: I was told by one mother that although she would have supported her son to die at home his siblings – already living independently – said they would feel unable to visit the family home if it had been the place of their brother's death. Such an 'ultimatum' places parents in an impossible situation, resulting in divided loyalties at a time of great stress.

Even when a home death is the preference of all concerned, an example from Ozzie, an eminent oncologist caring for TYAs with cancer, demonstrates that this is not always easy or manageable and may not always be the best option. The home can be turned into a replica of a hospital ward, and the 'through traffic' of visiting professionals can cause considerable disruption.

> A young girl who was I think about 19, with a younger brother who was doing his GCSEs, had quite a nasty end. And they made the downstairs through room ... [her] bedroom. And of course then, because she had all sorts of problems with paralysis and so on, and needing oxygen or whatever, the whole room was like a ward. And the nurses were coming in, and everybody was coming in ... although the GP wasn't, but that's another story. But how do they manage it? Because every time they came into the living room afterwards ... how do you escape that? It's very, very difficult.
> (Ozzie)

Ozzie raises the issue of continuing to live in the home after the death, yet in previous research I came across examples of families regarding their home as a 'shrine' after a death, creating 'sacred spaces' adorned with flowers and lighted candles (Grinyer and Thomas 2004). Indeed, it can become difficult for parents to leave a home that has been the place where their child has died. Nevertheless, it may be important to prepare families for the fact that their home will be taken over in this way. Ozzie also mentions the role of the GP: in this case the inference is that the GP's input was less than satisfactory. Vikky, a TCT nurse consultant emphasised the importance of the PTC liaising with the GP:

> I think we have a responsibility, as health professionals from the PTC, to ensure that a GP is informed and knowledgeable, and actually up to date with what's going on with their patients. And I think we need to be much more thoughtful about how you keep a GP involved, how you keep them up to date and how you keep them informed, so that ... when the focus of care shifts from hospital to home, the GP is in a better position to step in and help with that, rather than being kept on the outside and not being able to be involved. Again, one of the problems there of course, if you look about the delays in diagnosis, is that sometimes the family don't want that GP to be so actively involved. So you've got to find a way of overcoming that.
> (Vikky)

Interestingly, although there is a central role for a GP in supporting death at home (Vickers et al. 2007), and Anne spoke of how Ellen had trusted her GP and how supportive he had been in her final few weeks of life, and Val mentioned that a GP from her local practice was involved in Martin's end of life care; few participants spoke about their GPs. None told me they held any anger or resentment against their GP for misdiagnosis or delayed diagnosis – not uncommon in this age group (Engel 2005, Lewis 2005, Grinyer 2007a) – yet few talked about their contribution either. However, as Vikky suggests, effective communication and liaison between the PTC and the GP is essential for the support of a home death.

Discussion

The empirical data in this chapter allow us to make comparisons between the use of hospice services by the families of children with long-term complex life-limiting conditions and the young adults with cancer. They also allow us to compare the perceptions of professionals with those of users. Let us start by comparing the two distinct cohorts of users.

It is clear that the relationship between long-term users of hospice services and hospice staff is very different from that of families with a teenager or young adult with cancer and the hospice staff who support them. Since the birth of their children, many of the families of the long-term users have been accustomed to caring for their children, primarily in the home, with community-based support from hospice services and other sources. However, it appears to be the hospice services that understand best the needs of the children and offer the most support. Nevertheless, although these services are valued highly, they are limited and there are boundary issues relating to who should provide care in a crisis. This can lead to families gaining the impression that hospice staff feel they have been inappropriately called out and that under certain – largely undefined – circumstances, hospital services would have been more appropriately accessed. Thus, it seems that communications and resources are among the key issues for children's hospices in providing home care for this cohort. Palliative care for these children – which is not confined to the end of life stage, although this may be needed also – tends to be of lengthy duration, enabling a family to continue their care of the child with complex needs. The dependency that results from their need for hospice support may render the parents and families relatively 'powerless' The staff are gatekeepers to both the service and the service-user community and have the power to withhold support, thus to risk their disapprobation would be to risk 'membership' of the community and all that goes with it. Although there is no suggestion that such a threat is deliberate, it reflects a hierarchical structure shaped by those who hold the power. As a result there can be a tendency for parents to adopt a stance of 'grateful passivity' in response to a powerful staff in control of resources and much needed access to them (Grinyer, Payne and Barbarachild 2010).

Young adults with cancer face different challenges. There is firstly the question of whether home-based care and support is available locally. As we have seen, this age group –particularly between the ages of 16 and 18 – can fall through a gap in services that vary according to postcode. Despite the surprise of some community-based service managers when I asked about the lack of provision for 16–18-year-olds, this is not without precedent and is mentioned in the medical press. An article in the *BMJ* by the mother of Andrew, a young man of 17 dying from cancer, who could not get home-based care, offers an example:

> We discovered two things: one was that we live in a 'black hole' as far as community nursing was concerned – no community nursing covered our area. The second was that unbearable pain usually strikes in the middle of the night, with arrogant disregard for office hours.
> (Darnill and Gamage 2006: 1494)

Thus it seems that although it may not be 'common knowledge', particularly in regions where there is no lack of services for this age-band, this issue has been addressed in the public domain yet remains a problem in some locations. The result, as in Martin's case, can be distressing for the young person and the family as despite his eventual support from a variety of sources much anxiety accompanied the provision and organisation of his care. We have also seen there can be a problem for the over-18s when services are not 'joined-up' and transition from children's to adult services is not seamless. As Rosemarie said, an overlapping service, rather than joined-up services, would prevent young adults falling into the gap between them.

We have also seen that even where services exist, the additional training of staff is necessary in managing portacaths and Hickman lines and other technologies, if pain is to be managed reliably. The timely provision of drug therapies can be problematic but is essential if the child or young person is to be assured that their pain will not be allowed to get out of control. Where children's services are used, the professionals need to respect the relative maturity and life-stage of the adolescents and young adults they are caring for. Coordination of services can be achieved through shared care with the local hospital, hospice or other community services but this requires a degree of cooperation and collaboration that can be missing where professional boundaries become an issue or if the family have been advised against a home death.

Most participants felt that a home death allowed more control – that the family could organise itself with greater freedom around the domestic environment. Nevertheless, when the death is of a young person who is married, whether this is in the marital home or the parental home, issues of power and control become central. The gatekeeper in this setting is not the health professional but the mother-in-law or son- or daughter-in-law, which can exacerbate family tensions. It would be unrealistic to provide a formula for how such family dynamics might be addressed, but if professionals – and indeed family members – are aware that this is not unusual, it may allow for an open discussion and a strategy for setting aside differences during this difficult period. If, as we shall see in Chapter 5, the events surrounding the death affect the grieving process, it is of long-term importance that the death is managed as well as possible.

For families able to secure the support necessary for a home death, and whose family relationships remain harmonious, we have seen some very positive and meaningful experiences. Insofar as the death of a young person can ever be a 'good death', this can be achieved. Yet we have also seen that there can be unanticipated difficulties. For example, it seems that if a home death is to be managed in a way that does not leave family members traumatised, they need to be prepared for the bodily processes that lead up to death and also those that follow it. Bianca was unprepared for what the physical process of dying would entail; she repeatedly said that no one told her what it would be like, asking: 'Why did no-one explain it?'. Similarly, Beckie said: 'they won't talk about it', referring to preparing her for the physical manifestations of Billie's death. Likewise, Pat and her family were unprepared for the exudation of bodily fluids and rigor mortis; their preparation of Sara's body after death might have been a great deal less distressing had they known in advance about the physical processes that take place in the hours after death. These issues can be difficult for professionals to broach; it is hard enough to explain that a child or young person will die without having to detail the post mortem manifestations. Nevertheless, in cultures where death takes place mostly in hospice or hospital settings, and is thus managed mainly by professionals and 'out of sight', being prepared appears to be essential – particularly if the death takes place when no professionals are present.

Reference to siblings in the context of home death, although relatively sparse, suggests that each family is different; some families believed it to be beneficial for siblings for the death take place at home rather than in a clinical setting from which they may be excluded, whereas others felt having the death take place at home would be traumatic and unacceptable particularly for younger siblings. There was also a comment from a mother who said her adult children told her that they would have felt traumatised and unable to visit the family home if the death had taken place there. Some parents may also feel they cannot support a home death even if they have apparently accessed all the social and financial resources necessary. As Vikky commented:

> And also the individuality of some families ... I had one mum that would have liked to administer the subcut morphine herself ... if she had been allowed to, and probably previous to Harold Shipman [she] would have been ... but she couldn't do that ... she found that deeply troubling. For other parents, they don't want to have to be the nurse and the doctor; they want to be a mother ... Sometimes the burden of care, though the parents accept it, I think is so huge that actually I think especially when a child is dying, you don't want to have to always be the nurse and the doctor, you want to be mum or dad. And I think if we are going to advocate more successful deaths at home, that does have to come with a support package that truly is supportive and responsive to the needs of those parents, because it is them that the burden falls on.
> (Vikky)

Thus, it seems that each family is so individual that it is difficult to predict who will feel able to support a home death and who will not, but for those who do choose this option the accounts in this chapter should help professionals to understand what support is needed and what services are lacking, and for families to comprehend better what they are undertaking.

Lessons for best practice

Some of the above accounts tell stories of a good death achieved at home with the support of a wide range of professionals and well coordinated services, whereas others speak of distress above and beyond the terminal illness and death of a son or daughter. So what can we learn from the testimonies of both parents and professionals about what is needed to achieve the best experience under such distressing circumstances? The following points are suggestions for changing policy and improving practice:

- Reliable community-based services available 24 hours a day and at weekends are needed for the peace of mind and security of the family and their son or daughter
- Such services should not be dependent on a 'postcode lottery' - which seems particularly to be the case for 16–18-year-olds
- These services must be provided by professionals skilled and familiar with the latest technology to support end of life care and appropriate palliative treatment

- The provision of pain-relief drugs must be rapid and reliable
- Where several services are involved, coordination between them is essential and parents must be clear about who to call on for what service
- It must be clear exactly what home-based services can offer, and if and when hospital admission may be appropriate, particularly when palliative care is delivered over a lengthy period for chronic illness
- If the patient is a teenager or young adult, the professionals delivering the services must also be aware that an age-appropriate approach is essential if the TYA is not to feel patronised
- Families need to be prepared for what to expect of the physical processes that accompany death and for the post-death bodily manifestations
- There should be better recognition that not all families are prepared for what a home death entails and may be in need of unanticipated medical and social support
- Some family circumstances can be complicated, and where power struggles are apparent sensitivity is needed, and the introduction of counselling or other support services may be appropriate
- After the death, a house previously filled with professionals and activity may feel desolate and the family can feel abandoned, so follow-up support is important in the immediate aftermath of the death and possibly for some time later

Chapter 3
Hospice-based Palliative and End of Life Care

The first children's hospice, opened in Oxford in 1982, Helen House was groundbreaking at that time and has served as a model for most of the children's hospices subsequently developed in the UK (Price and McFarlane 2009). There are currently 44 children's hospice services in the UK (ACT 2009) providing support for children with complex and life-limiting conditions and their families. As the ACT document states, the provision of short breaks offered in a variety of forms by these services is enormously beneficial for the whole family, providing much-needed respite from care to parents and carers and a welcome break for the child. The range of services may include: inpatient hospice care; hospice at home; sitting services; befriender/activity services; short break fostering; community houses and domiciliary care (ACT 2009: 14). However, according to Brown and Warr (2007: 21), paediatric palliative care is still very patchy in its provision, there is no national plan and children's hospices tend to spring up where local individuals have had the 'finance, charisma or drive to make it happen'.

As Price and McFarlane (2009) point out, it is a commonly held misconception that children's hospices provide end of life care for children with cancer, but this is not usually the case as children with malignancies rarely use hospice care. The children cared for in children's hospices tend not to be acute cases but to have long-term complex and chronic illnesses, and may receive palliative care for many years throughout their infancy, childhood and adolescence. However, although children's hospices provide long term-palliative care they can also provide end of life care as necessary.

Pfund (2007) points out that not all children's hospices offer care to adolescents and young adults. Indeed, the upper age limit in Northern Ireland is 10 years old, whereas in the rest of the UK there is what Pfund describes as a two-tier system whereby 18-year-olds with a new diagnosis are not eligible for services that would be offered to 18-year-olds with a long-standing diagnosis. According to Pfund:

> If a young person has DMD (Duchenne Muscular Dystrophy) and is referred to a children's hospice while under the age of 16 years, he is

Palliative and End of Life Care for Children and Young People: Home, Hospice and Hospital, First Edition. Anne Grinyer.
© 2012 John Wiley & Sons, Ltd. Published 2012 by John Wiley & Sons, Ltd.

accepted under category 2, and depending on the age limit up to which the hospice is licensed, he can access its services for the rest of his life. However, if a referral is not made until he is 18 years of age, the same young man cannot be accepted into children's hospice care.
(Pfund 2007: 99–100)

This can mean that newly diagnosed adolescents – for example those with cancers – can fall between services. Whether or not an 18-year-old in this situation would actually want to be cared for in a paediatric hospice environment is another matter, which is discussed later in this chapter.

Craig (2006) says transition from paediatric to adult services can be extremely difficult for young people and their families, so the provision of an intermediate adolescent option would appear to make sense. According to Pfund (2007: 99), Martin House in Yorkshire takes young people up to the age of 31, but in an interview with their Head of Care it became apparent that they will in fact care for young adults up to the age of 35 but will accept no new admissions over the age of 19 unless their life expectancy appears to be very short. Pfund says that Douglas House in Oxford takes young people up to the age of 40 but again an interview with their Head of Care suggests that their lower age limit is 16 and their upper limit 35. Other adolescent hospice provision is being planned and some adolescent wings or annexes are being developed for both children's and adult hospices. (Interviews with some of those developing these initiatives are included in the *Findings* below). There is no doubt that such developments are to be welcomed, but the research findings discussed below demonstrate that for young adults with cancer these care settings, although designed for the age group, may still present challenges to teenagers and young adults (TYAs) – particularly those with cancer – and in some instances to the staff.

The other hospice-based alternative is adult care, but as Pfund (2007) says, the model for adult hospice care does not necessarily meet the needs of young people. Adult hospices tend to provide end of life care in the immediate period before death, usually up to 2 weeks. In contrast, the model for children's respite care is of block weeks over an extended period of years. Thus, this model of care may be problematic for the children with complex and life-limiting conditions familiar with paediatric care and for young adults with cancer to whom the care setting may appear unacceptable.

The children who use children's hospice services tend to be those with complex and life-limiting conditions, with which they have been born or which have developed in early childhood, rather than childhood cancers. Craig (2006) argues that caring for a child with a life-limiting illness, particularly if there are physical limitations and deteriorating health, places an immense demand on parents. Thus, she says, it is important that there should be the provision of inpatient respite care for scheduled breaks and emergencies. Taking a children's hospice service as a case study example, the first part of the 'findings' draws on empirical data gathered from users, in an attempt to understand how the services are experienced, what the limitations are, how the hospice service relates to other sources of support and how well the transition from paediatric to adult services is managed. The data, which are intended to provide a glimpse of what it is like to be a family caring for a child with complex life-limiting illness using hospice palliative care services, consider the issues raised by the participants using illustrative quotes. The extended nature of palliative care for these children means their longer-term needs and transition issues are also the focus of discussion. The hospice services addressed in this chapter relate to inpatient care, as home-based support was included in the previous chapter.

Readers will note that there is a distinctive difference in the sources of empirical data in the remainder of this chapter. The majority of the participants in the children's hospice discussion are the users; there is little published material on how these services are experienced by parents and children, whose firsthand accounts are focused on here. The families who use children's hospice services tend to be long-term users, very grateful for the support they receive and reluctant to voice any criticism lest they seem ungrateful; thus, their voices and experiences remain unheard. In contrast, the majority of the material drawn on in the discussion of TYAs with cancer comes from hospice service providers. As shown in the tables in Chapter 1, there are currently relatively few TYAs with cancer using hospice services; as a consequence, there are few accounts of the use of such services by this cohort. However, there is a growing commitment in the hospice movement to extend services that will be attractive to them. Their struggles in achieving this aim are documented here – again through firsthand accounts, which tend not to be documented elsewhere.

Nonetheless, there is an area of overlap between the two cohorts – the transition from paediatric to adult services – which connects the two parts of the chapter. Furthermore, bringing together the data gathered from my studies with both cohorts allows for an element of comparison between the differing needs and expectations of the users in each case. Thus, the dilemma for the 'hospice movement' as a whole can be seen in the context of the sometimes contrasting and competing demands for their services.

Findings

Children with complex and life-limiting conditions

The physical needs of the children included in this study were many and varied but all had complex, multiple and profound physical and cognitive impairments that required a great deal of management. The importance of an inpatient respite service in sustaining the ongoing support given by parents was summed up by Lily as she described the physical struggle entailed in caring for her daughter Karen, aged 21:

> Karen has severe cerebral palsy, and has many complex nursing needs. She has epilepsy, scoliosis and pressure sores and cannot function at all

> by herself; she has no movement and cannot speak, but can vocalise, and talks with her eyes. Over the last 7 or 8 years, her needs have increased: her spine has now collapsed [and] one of her lungs, so she functions on about 60% lung capacity, giving rise to more chest infections, and pneumonia … For the last 3 years we have to take oxygen wherever we go, suction machines, nebulisers. She is on two different medications for her chest, which are taken daily to help prevent the amount of chest infections. Obviously she has grown, which makes things more difficult, because I am not overly big.
> (Lily)

Karen's range of needs are typical of those found in the study, all the children from infants upwards had multiple and complex conditions necessitating constant input from the family – the only real respite is inpatient palliative care. However, as the children become older and bigger, the physical demands on parents increase, as Lily mentioned in her account. As support for such needs may not always be found through primary care services, hospice care is relied on as an essential source of support and advice as Brenda, Matthew's mother, indicated:

> Advice and support when Matthew went from oral eating to being tube-fed [from the hospice] … was invaluable. The staff would sit with me while the dietician went through everything … My GP never really got to know Matthew or about his condition – the hospice have supported me.
> (Brenda)

It seems that the expertise of hospice staff and the amount of time they are able to put in to the support of such children is in contrast to the busy GP, who is not only not an expert in what may be a very rare condition – in this case Miller-Dieker syndrome – a rare genetic disorder but who may not have the time or resources to engage to the same extent as the staff in the hospice. As ACT (2011d) say, many GPs may only care for one or two children with life-limiting conditions in their entire working life. Thus, the hospice has a key role not only in the relief of the 'care burden', but also in the appropriate management of the condition.

Yet despite the obvious benefits derived from hospice support, there may be barriers and disincentives to the use of more routine inpatient services. For example, there may be little choice over when respite care is offered, it may not coincide with the families' preferences or fit with their plans but instead has to be taken as and when it is available. Accessing the hospice may also be problematic, Tania raised the issue of support with transport; living 10 miles from the hospice meant the practicalities of taking her son Dan for respite care were challenging:

> It just would have been great if they could have offered a transport service to and from, that would make life easier … on your own with him in the car …

if he was having a fit in the car or needing oxygen, I would be driving and I would have to pull over. I have pulled over on the motorway before now. I have had to call an ambulance to the side of the road, and things like that. In those situations it would have been really good if I had had some-one from the hospice who could come for him and I would know he was safe or to travel with us. That would have been a real improvement. (Tania)

Inpatient respite care is greatly valued but for what might sometimes be perceived as minimal provision – many inpatient respite visits were no more than 2 or 3 days long – the amount of paperwork was thought to make it almost not worth the trouble. For example according to Nancy: 'Sometimes it's more hassle than it's worth, filling in all the forms etc ... it's a lot of paper-work and once a year there's an extensive care-plan to fill in'. A similar comment was made by Dan's stepmother, Tania, who said there was too much form filling for each visit. She added that when Dan went for day care it was: 'Very difficult, packing up everything just for the day – almost not worth the bother'.

Such comments suggest that although, as we have seen, inpatient respite care is a lifeline, it comes at a price – if the lack of choice and the amount of advance organisation required is accompanied by bureaucracy on arrival for a relatively short visit, families may question the extent to which the benefit outweighs the cost.

When to use the hospice service

The needs of the children and of their parents who use inpatient hospice palliative care services are not consistent or predictable and there may be points in the illness trajectory that trigger crises requiring an urgent response. Yet although such pressing needs are generally met, some comments implied that whereas hospice support could not be faulted in terms of emergency input, unless there was an urgent need, families felt they had to cope them-selves with the 'everyday' demands of their child's condition. For example, although knowing that the hospice staff were only a phone call away was of importance to Leo's guardian Una, she had uncertainties about her 'right' to use it: 'It's busy [there] and really for terminally ill children. If I have a problem, I'll sort it out by myself' (Una).

Given what we have seen in the literature about children's hospices not primarily being for 'terminally ill' children but for long-term palliative support, this response is perhaps surprising but was also echoed by others. A similar observation was made by baby Barnie's mother Susan who voiced her reservations about non-emergency provision: 'They're always good in an emergency ... very good with palliative care ... but then when it is all going right, I sometimes find them not very helpful. You know, for us to get on with it, sort of thing'. Although she would have taken Barnie to hospital in an acute crisis, Susan said that if he was fitting, or needed a drip she would take him to the hospice, but she added, 'I think he has to be on death's door, sort of thing, that's what it seems like to us' (Susan).

Although some parents felt they could not prevail on the hospice for 'everyday' needs, others were concerned that taking a 'poorly' child to the hospice was not acceptable. As Tess's mother Nancy said:

> In the past when we have used it, they have had the doctor in to listen to her chest and said she has got a chest infection or she has got a throat infection, but I wouldn't knowingly take her [to the hospice] poorly.
> (Nancy)

Sheila, the Head of Care at a children's/adolescent hospice, reflected on the confusion and uncertainty about when it is appropriate to seek inpatient hospice care and when it is more appropriate to take the child to hospital:

> A lot of the children have a dress rehearsal of death a number of times ... I think that is one of the difficulties for a lot of the parents who use us ... which is why the death rate ... in hospital is often higher ... Families ... would often go to the hospital as the first line of action and then unfortunately the child may die on that occasion. So, one of the things that we are looking at is end of life care plans, or care plans around which treatment options are now viable. I think often that's quite ironed out in oncology that we can't give any more active treatment, we're not going to do this or we are going to do that ... Whereas, often, in the other conditions the children have had lots of events that have led them into hospital in an acute phase. But, at some point, you're trying to look at when is it right to go into hospital or when is it not, which is when you would write up a care plan.
> (Sheila)

Sheila's comments echo the literature in emphasising how difficult it may be to predict the point at which palliative care becomes end of life care and the importance of drawing up a care plan. She also pointed out the importance of the circumstances of extubation when the expectation would be that the child would die as a result, although she said that this is not always the case:

> What you plan to do is to make it a much nicer environment and less stressful, where the family can be alongside without another little child on the bed next door. But it's also looking at the longer picture ... if they do survive ... but ... most probably wouldn't, and then would maybe use our facilities for sort of aftercare once the child had died as well. But that is something that quite a number of hospices are doing in a nicer environment. And I think, sort of recently this year, we've had occasions where babies have been born and never got out of a unit. And to actually come with the grounds and things, for the parents it's lovely that they

feel they've had some fresh air. It's something that's really valuable ... And even just a simple thing like the fresh air coming through the room is something that they want their baby to have experienced.
(Sheila)

So it seems that the acute physical needs of the patients are recognised and largely met by the hospice services, and that this is valued highly, particularly as it appears that such needs are in some cases not well understood by primary care services. Nevertheless, there was an indication that in addition to the challenges of actually reaching the hospice with a very disabled child, parents can feel their son or daughter's 'everyday' needs are their responsibility and that unless there is an emergency it is up to the family to provide the support and care. However, there is also the example of the family who would never knowingly take their daughter to the hospice when 'poorly'. Although it was not specified whether this was in order to prevent introduction of infection, this indicates differing perceptions of what the hospice is able and willing to provide in terms of physical care and when it is appropriate to expect inpatient services.

The criticisms voiced by the parents relating to the availability of respite care, transport difficulties and the level of bureaucracy raise the question of how much it is reasonable to expect in terms of support. In order to establish how services are organised elsewhere, I undertook an interview with Clare, the Director of Clinical Services at a renowned and well-established children's hospice. It was clear from her responses that although a slightly different model is in operation, there are nevertheless limits to what can be offered. She told me that each family is allocated a certain number of nights of inpatient respite care; this varies from 10 to 28 nights per year depending on the family's need and how much additional help they receive from other sources. It is up to the families to make their bookings, but half their stays have to be outside the peak times of school holidays and weekends. No more than three stays can be booked in advance to give everyone a chance, and a family taking 2 weeks in August in one year is unlikely be allocated the same the following year. Nevertheless, despite the finite number of beds, the hospice staff are flexible enough to be able to respond to emergencies, so if a parent contacts them and says that they are at the end of their tether, they will accommodate the child on an emergency basis. Clearly, there is a limit to how many children could be offered such care at any one time, but the impression was that this is a self-regulating system that works well. There is no routine offer of help with transport but if a family was struggling there would be an attempt to support them – perhaps by advocating on their behalf with their local authority. The paperwork would also be streamlined so that it was not an onerous task on arrival, and if nothing had changed since the previous visit there would simply be a check that the necessary drugs were available, and the doctor would ask the parents if there was anything that needed to be discussed. Parents seemed to be empowered by participating in a parents' user group, a Facebook page for parents and a parent-run bereavement group for other more recently bereaved parents. What is apparent here is that, despite finite resources, there is a degree of flexibility and responsiveness to the individual needs of parents.

End of life care

Although most of the families interviewed had not been bereaved, it nevertheless became apparent that end of life care is a crucial element of the support provided by the hospice and is anticipated as a possible future need by some families. However, there was no indication in any instance that end of life decisions had been shared with the young person, and in this sample it may be primarily because the children in question were very young or had cognitive impairments (this issue is discussed further in Chapter 5).

Families may have different preferences relating to end of life care and place of death. However, the importance of support from the hospice was expressed by Tania, the stepmother of Dan, who died aged 16: 'Six months before his death, the respite was such a lifeline – to be normal for 2 or 3 days. They were very supportive of me and the kids' (Tania). However, Tania's younger son, Nick, 5 at the time of Dan's death, had after the death, been in urgent need of counselling, which was not available until a few months later. This suggests that siblings may be in need of support in the immediate aftermath of a death, when the family are in shock and grieving and when the familiarity of the staff and environment at the hospice may have been 'lost' to them abruptly (there is a more detailed discussion of bereavement needs in Chapter 5).

Len and Diane had fostered many children with complex needs, ten of whom had used the hospice services and three of whom had died. This family said that they could not have undertaken their foster care of children with disabilities without the support they received from the hospice and said the following: 'We've lost three boys – we wouldn't have missed a minute – but we couldn't have done it without them [the hospice]' (Len). The hospice helped Diane and Len to manage a home death for the first of their foster children who died, visiting every day and eventually going to the funeral home with them. The deceased second and third children went directly to the hospice following their deaths in the hospital. Asked what happened toward the end of the children's lives, Len said: 'They came immediately they heard. A member of the nursing staff would come even on her day off'. Even though the deaths took place in their home and at the hospital, the hospice staff were nevertheless closely involved and supported the family not only throughout the end of life phase but also after their deaths. As Diane said: 'None of the three children have died at the hospice, but they have helped us with training for caring ... [and bereavement counselling] for all the children who died' (Diane). However, not all families need the same type of support after a death; the guardian of one the hospice users said: 'I knew bereavement counselling was available, but we haven't needed it – even though I lost my brother 6 months ago' (Una) (see also Chapter 5).

As we have seen, palliative care for children with life-limiting conditions can extend across many years and it may be difficult to predict when the end of life phase will begin. Most parents did not want to engage in discussion about end of life care plans – perhaps because talking about it may make it appear to be more of a reality or even to expedite it. Nevertheless, there was a suggestion from some parents that it was important to maintain contact with the hospice as a kind of 'insurance policy' against a future implicit need for it to be a place where end of life care could be offered. Some parents whose children no longer used the hospice service as much as they had in the past (like Leo) still valued the links. Una, Leo's guardian, said she was happy for Leo to still have regular contact with the hospice, in case of 'future eventualities'.

Planning for change – transition issues

If we take the wider definition of palliative care as being the relief of pain and suffering and offering a support system to both the patient and their family (Clark and Wright 2003), then it is clear that this care can extend across a considerable period of time, necessitating changes in the type and location of provision. The issue of planning for the nature of the care to change was, according to most parents, handled with sensitivity. Martha, the mother of 8-year-old Mandy, spoke about the likelihood of future overnight visits for her daughter and the gradual way she was introduced to the experience:

> After January ... we are going to start trying Martha sleeping over once a week ... The staff have been introducing her to the bedrooms and saying she can have 'High School Musical' [duvet] covers on, she would be able to have a little nap and watch telly. The thing they are trying to do at the moment is get Martha confident with the night staff, the people that are there and the children that are there, just to make it more easy for Martha ... we need to set things in place now, so in the long run it is not going to be too distressing for her.
> (Mandy)

Although relatively short-term plans were of importance, some parents had longer-term concerns. Nancy was anxious about what might happen when the hospice could no longer care for Tess after she reached the age of 30. Sharon, whose son Edward was 18 and approaching the end of his entitlement to children's services, was concerned about the provision of his health care once he left the hospice and said: 'Nothing's set in concrete – we have to be very flexible – and the one thing [Social Services] don't grasp is, you need a set plan. This is unacceptable - but it seems to be the norm' (Sharon). Although Sharon is critical of Social Services, there is perhaps a role here for the hospice staff to help smooth the transition process. There is some evidence that this is happening. Nadia said her family had been contacted about transition for Karl at nearly 15, although it seems she was unclear about why this was being broached:

> Somebody has rung recently, they are coming out to talk to us about transition ... they want to talk to us about transition but I don't really understand why, so I might ring them before they come and say why, because I am not any use going to meetings unprepared.
> (Nadia)

Although Nadia, whose son was only 15, had been approached about transition and appeared not to understand why, parents of older service users were concerned that there had been no planning for their longer-term future. Karen's mother, Lily, expressed anxiety about the next stage for her daughter Karen at 21: 'It goes from getting it all to nothing at all ... it's absolutely preposterous' (Lily)

It seems there is some discrepancy here in the understanding of how long long-term service users can go on using a paediatric hospice: there was concern for Tess after she turned 30, whereas at only 18 Edward's mother was already worried, as was Karen's mother at 21. Melissa indicated she had no idea how long her daughter Hannah would be entitled to care at the hospice and although Hannah was only 4 and a half, Melissa was already expressing concern:

> I do worry about the future and what she will be like as an adult. I have been worrying about what would happen when I am elderly and what would happen to her, or when one of us dies, I don't know. There is no family, his [husband's] family don't live around here and my mum died last year, so I only have my dad, but my dad doesn't really have the patience for her and she is hard work and he is in his 60s and can't deal with it. I just worry about where she will go, one day it might happen ... I haven't talked to them about it. I don't know what they do beyond the age of 18, is it 18 they go there?
> (Melissa)

Although some of these concerns relate to services available outside the hospice provision, there is clearly an element of anxiety about planning for a future without the hospice. The sense of being abandoned by a service they have come to trust and rely on, with apparently no idea of what will follow, was summed up by Lily who said: 'there doesn't seem to be anything out there for the older sector'. Although, clearly, other services are available, they seem to be perceived as only a vague concept. Lily had identified a possible provider of care for Karen after she leaves the hospice but her anxiety and difficulty in entrusting others with her care is clear from the following quote:

> Losing the hospice this year will be a nightmare. We need respite which offers everything they can offer. I haven't ruled out Karen living in the community by herself – but I don't trust anyone with my kids ...
> (Lily)

Some of Lily's concern may be because living outside the immediate catchment area of the hospice she was uncertain if Karen would be entitled to continuing services. Nevertheless, there was an indication from a number of participants that in the long term, there was a considerable amount of anxiety about 'what happens next' – what care provision would be available when the young people became too old for the children's hospice services.

Although moving on to adult care may be a concern, there was recognition that the older children were outgrowing the child-orientated setting. The children's hospice play facilities were used by both the patients and their siblings, but there were observations that because the age range of the children using the facilities was wide, the presence and noise of the younger children could be problematic for the older children. Martha's mother Mandy said Martha didn't like it when the babies cried – which at only 8 is a remarkably similar response to those of the older children (see below). Brenda made a similar observation about the play facilities: '[we need] more for teenagers – the play area is lovely, but is focused on the smaller children' (Brenda).

The hospice in this case study will support young people up to the age of 30. Other children's hospices may vary in their upper age limit but there was concern about age-appropriate care at the upper end of the hospice's age range. For example, Tess was 26, and had multiple physical impairments and attended a day care centre for adults with learning disabilities 4 days a week. However, she also spent 1 day a month at the hospice. Her mother, Nancy, spoke with both gratitude and ambivalence about Tess's use of the hospice services as Tess, who started at the hospice in 1996 aged 14, enjoyed some aspects of the hospice but found others challenging:

> It's not her favourite place – but she doesn't panic when we go there … She enjoys the social side of the hospice: the big plasma screen TV, the craft room, and dinner! But she doesn't like the children crying and screaming.
> (Nancy)

Nancy suggested that there should be an adolescent unit off the lounge – as she said: 'Not so much of the tinies'. Nancy thought that the hospice had missed an opportunity to put resources into developing adolescent care, which a young person of Tess's age would have valued:

> I just think it's a shame that they did massive fundraising a few years ago and they did very little to improve the hospice, when you consider the amount of money they raised. I mean that big admin building popped up, and I think that's where most of the money went, I think that's a bit naughty really, when it was all fundraised for the hospice, but they did make some improvement, the computer room is an add-on, but they didn't put any more bedrooms in … Some of the other children's hospices are now creating adolescent units, and I think maybe it is something they [the hospice] could have considered.
> (Nancy)

Tess's care worker, Rory, reiterated the importance of age-appropriate care:

> Age-appropriate can have many different meanings. For example, Tess enjoys children's TV – which she couldn't ... in Social Services respite ... It's important to treat Tess as an individual. [When Tess stays at the hospice] she can use the communal lounge and the sensory room, and has her own bedroom. The main lounge is noisy, so I take her to her bedroom, where she can relax with the TV and the DVD player.
> (Rory)

There was an assumption that the focus of the hospice was on younger children and that this could affect attitudes to young adult users. As Nancy said: 'As a mum, when I go to the hospice, the staff and volunteers make a bee-line for the little ones, fuss the babies – don't come over to Tess. [My husband] said, "Tess has had her time"' (Nancy). Tess's care worker added: 'Staff work [at the hospice] *because* it's a children's hospice' (Rory), thus implying that staff have a greater interest in the younger children.

Related to concerns about age-appropriate care was the worry about what happens when the young person reaches an age when the hospice can no longer offer support. A number of parents admitted to being worried about the future and anxious about the type of care their child would be offered. Although Nancy is concerned about what will happen when the hospice can no longer care for Tess after she reaches the age of 30, this issue can be managed with skill, as when Brenda described how, with advance planning, her son Matthew was transferred into a residential care setting. Matthew's transition from children's to adult care provision began when he was 14, with the guidance and support of a PCT [primary care trust] Transition Officer. As Brenda said: 'You want [your children] to move on – I wanted [him] to have that experience' (Brenda). This example demonstrates that when care planning is undertaken in advance in liaison with other services, it can work well for all concerned and alleviate the anxiety caused by the transitional process.

The rationale for setting up an adolescent annexe to an existing children's hospice was provided by Sheila, Head of Care at what became a combined children's/young adult hospice:

> We'd thought about it for a number of years ... a lot of the children were surviving into young adulthood, into their teenage years, which previously hadn't happened, and were really wanting something different. For the majority of children who use us, independence is quite hard to achieve, and we felt that they wanted something where they could experience independence, look at the boundaries, be more adult, have more choices, and I think, have a flexible environment that enabled them to do all of those things. Because a number of them are very dependent on their families ... it's trying to give them a break ... which, as an adolescent, is something that you really want to do ... Initially, when we opened the teenage unit, it was the very articulate young people who could have

a very open choice about whether they wanted to go over there and try it or not. But gradually, some of the young people with more complex care [needs] have moved over and it's been wonderful to see the way in which they've grown.
(Sheila)

However, an interview with Rosemarie, a Senior Palliative Care Nurse Specialist at an adult hospice working with the adult home care team, raised a number of issues about decision making once young people, particularly those with learning difficulties, become adult:

And that's sort of one of the big things I think that came out of the ... patients who came through from the children's services, was this shift of power, which is very difficult for a parent, especially if the young person has got a learning disability or, you know, maybe emotionally isn't able to cope with, you know, their disease. And the parents, you know, naturally the power falls to them, but legally we have to sort of defer to the young adult. And if they've got capacity then that's what we have to do. So quite often you find yourself sort of being a bit of a negotiator and it can be very difficult. And you know and we're not even talking just the sort of 18-year-olds, but quite often the young adults are in their mid-twenties. They still live at home ... you know, they've been used to parents making all the big decisions, you know, run the house – they just have to get up and do their life. They don't have to make these decisions and all of a sudden, you know, people are asking them to make huge decisions, which they've never had to do.
(Rosemarie)

So it seems not only do the children have to manage a transition – so do their parents. This can be a problem for young adults who do not have cognitive disabilities, but for those who do the shift of power referred to by Rosemarie can be even more problematic. Hospices can play a key role here in supporting the change needed in the family dynamics to allow the young people to live as autonomously as possible for the remainder of their lives and enable the parents to shift the balance of power as appropriate.

Hospice care for TYAs with cancer

We can see that even for the young people who have been cared for in a paediatric hospice environment for most of their lives, when they reach adolescence they begin to feel out of place. Yet, as became clear from responses to the Teenage Cancer Trust (TCT) end of life care service evaluation (Grinyer and Barbarachild 2011), adult hospices do not necessarily offer an acceptable alternative. As one occupational therapist said: 'If they are offered a place in an adult hospice, it can be a complete nightmare'. The challenge of offering appropriate hospice care for TYAs was summarised by Sarah, the Director of Nursing at an adolescent hospice:

> ... [children's hospices] are fantastic places. Predominantly they care for children and young adults with non-cancer conditions. The cancer patients tend to obviously go to the adult hospices, so there is this awful gap at the moment in the middle. You know, where do the young adults go, where do they actually sit comfortably? Young adults ... want to play their music loud; they want to watch DVDs and the television into the early hours of the morning. They might want to go out and socialise with their friends. And just because they're ill, just because they've got a cancer diagnosis, or perhaps because they know they're terminal, it doesn't mean that they're going to give up on all those things at all. If anything it's going to make them more anxious to want to do those things.
> (Sarah)

Ozzie, a retired Professor of Adolescent Oncology, summed up the problem as follows:

> We do find it's very difficult indeed to get people admitted. Each [children's] hospice ... is very quirky ... although they pay lip service ... they really don't take above 16, although they said they would extend it, but I haven't seen any evidence of that. Occasionally you can force a patient in. But they're quite quirky in whether they take people or not – if they know them and ... most of their patients are not cancer patients. [This hospice] is superb ... they are very good. But again ... they do have sort of limits ... just because they're very busy and they take a lot of patients. And adult ones were very unwilling to take anybody under 18, so that middle age – you know, the sort of 16 to 18 – is quite difficult.
> (Ozzie)

So we can see that professionals working with TYAs are well aware of the issues relating to finding suitable hospice provision that the young people will feel is appropriate and that the hospices will be able to provide within their remit. The discussion now turns to a consideration of different hospice settings and the challenges they face in offering appropriate care for TYAs with cancer. Each sector, paediatric, adult and adolescent/young adult, will be discussed in turn, to consider their ability to provide for this age group with cancer, which tends to fall between care providers.

Children's hospice care

The need, expressed by the long-term users of the children's hospice, for a more age-appropriate care setting indicates that familiarity is not enough for users to remain satisfied with an environment they have outgrown. If this is problematic for the young people to whom the care setting is very familiar, the situation for the teenager or young adult who is suddenly diagnosed with a life-threatening condition such as cancer may be even more challenging. Most children's hospices do not care for many children with cancer, although one children's hospice happened to be caring for two children with cancer at the time of my visit, a 4-year-old and a 15-year-old. However, they said this was very unusual as the primary treatment centre (PTC) will normally continue their care until late in the illness, at which point the parents usually prefer to take their child home. However, there are exceptions to this model of care; another children's hospice I visited had a special relationship with a large regional hospital that cared for young adults with cancer, which resulted in a higher than usual number of young people with cancer between the ages of 16 and 24 being referred to the hospice for end of life care. Although some of those young people agreed to investigate the possibility of care in this children's hospice, they did not all agree to become inpatients. Despite a specially designated adolescent room, excellent facilities and welcoming staff, the young adults disliked the child-orientated décor and found it difficult to identify with the young hospice users whose medical conditions and complex needs were unfamiliar to them. As a result they refused to be cared for in this environment, leaving their families to find an alternative. Elaine, the Head of Clinical Services at a children's hospice, encapsulates the issues:

We would accept, if there was a child ... young person, should I say? ... coming towards the end of their life [if] they were 19 or 20 ... Of course then we need to be certain that this is the right environment for that young person. And they've got choices to make as well. And one of the challenges, really, is that although we try and make the environment suitable for all age groups, as you walk in you probably notice ... it leans towards the younger age group, with the number of fluffy toys and things around. We've had young people that have used our service here for end of life care ... and it wasn't their first choice. Their first choice would have been to be at home, but because of the physical environment in which they live [it] wasn't suitable to meet their care needs ... they might have lived in a flat where there were steps to get up to it, and [if] they've got mobility requirements ... it wasn't suitable for them to be at home, so they were here. It may be that it's a parental choice. Although young people are able to make decisions for themselves, particularly post-16, if family members feel unable to support them in their choices then sometimes that is still taken out of their hands.

I remember one young person of 16 that was referred to our service and had quite an aggressive tumour and was obviously coming towards the end of their life, and they came to see the service here, because the family felt that they couldn't care for the young person at home. And she felt that this environment wasn't right for her. The family felt that it was right, but she didn't ... I think because ... on the day she visited the number of children with very complex disabilities that were here. And I mean she was obviously a young person and quite able, and ... she didn't feel that that was the right place for her, so she chose to die in hospital ... [despite the fact that] one of our rooms is very specifically teenagery,

> with an en-suite bathroom and everything. So she could have had that as her room. She actually wouldn't have needed to communicate with anyone else if she didn't want to. She could have just used that facility … But she agreed that after her death that her body could come here to our special bedroom, and the family took on that support. So that was her choice, but … if there had been an annexe here or an annexe or at an adult hospice that was specifically for teenagers, I suspect she would have opted for that. And that may have been the most suitable place for her. The family … actually had a young sibling in the family, and this environment, with lots of toys, would have been ideal for the sibling. So if you had a teenage annexe with similar facilities for siblings, then that would have been a fantastic opportunity.
>
> (Elaine)

Not only may the adolescent patient be resistant to a children's care setting, the staff may also be unused to caring for acute illness in the age group. Although emergency admissions may take place and deaths do occur, some staff at children's hospices may not be as used to deaths as might be expected as the care tends to be for long-term chronic conditions during short bouts of respite care. There may also be a lack of clinical expertise in the management of cancer-related illness, and unfamiliarity with the drug regimes and the aggressive nature of acute illness in previously healthy young people, which can manifest itself in distressing ways. Vikky, a Nurse Consultant for the TCT said of children's hospice care for oncology patients:

> Some of the care that can be delivered in a children's hospice doesn't meet the needs of the child dying [of cancer] … they can't do blood products, they can't do some of the other stuff, just because the care's different. It's not a criticism; it's just that it's different.
> (Vikky)

This is acknowledged in Liz's comments about her work at Helen House Children's Hospice before she was instrumental in setting up Douglas House Hospice for Young Adults:

> Teenagers and young adults with cancer are quite a specific group, in that the cancers that they have behave differently from either childhood cancers or from the cancers which affect older adults. There is a growing body of research that is showing that actually the disease process is different. And I felt that given that there was this growing recognition, and also some of the cancers that are most common for this age group can be quite aggressive cancers, and therefore treatment success rates are poorer for the teenage and young adult population than they are for the paediatric population. So I was very aware that there was this

growing awareness that the disease process is different and also that
the success of treatment is maybe not as high as it is in children.
(Liz)

Thus, we can see that even if a children's hospice has some expertise in
supporting children with cancer – which does not constitute their main
caseload – they may still be challenged by the clinical care of a TYA with
cancer. And if the patient has come from a TCT unit, designed around the
adolescent life stage, their expectations may challenge staff. Staying in bed
late in the morning, being up late at night or having a boyfriend or girlfriend
in their room, perhaps even overnight, may all be unfamiliar to paediatric
staff. However, Elaine, Head of Clinical Services at a children's hospice, said it
would be acceptable if a young person's partner wanted to stay overnight if
they were over 18, but the situation would have to be handled with sensitivity.
It is interesting that Elaine specified 'over 18' as the age at which a sexual
relationship is permissible in the hospice, as the age of consent is 16. Whether
at 16 or 18, young people's sexual activity usually remains hidden from their
parents' view, and certainly from the view of their health professionals, so
many adjustments and individual judgements would need to be made, and
some paediatric staff will inevitably find condoning and facilitating such
activity difficult. Paediatric staff tend to have chosen to work with children
rather than adolescents, whose behaviours may be experienced as challenging
and whose use of the services – as we have seen – will differ considerably
both medically and socially from that of children with complex life-limiting
illness with whom the staff are much more familiar.

Adult hospices

The most readily available alternative to children's hospice provision is
normally to be found at an adult hospice. Although it is unusual for an adult
hospice to be asked to accept a young person with a chronic life-limiting
condition, who will be more likely to stay on for care in a children's setting,
young adults diagnosed with acute and life-threatening illness may seek end
of life care at an adult hospice. However, adult hospices are not usually able to
accept young people under the age of 18 because this is not covered in their
licence. To negotiate agreement for exceptions requires that the Care Quality
Commission (CQC) local inspectorate agree. To be satisfied that facilities are
in place for a person under 18 in an adult hospice, the hospice may have to
demonstrate, for example, that if necessary they would be able to handle the
body appropriately. The director of one adult hospice said 'we can't put
them in the same fridge as an old person'. He was unable to explain why, even
if the young person and their family had no objections in principle, other
than that this was the regulation. His assumption may be unfounded, but it is
interesting evidence of the uncertainty about the appropriateness of
procedures relating to young people.

In some cases, if the CQC inspector agrees that there are appropriate
measures in place to support a person under 18, approval can be granted

rapidly on the telephone and admission can take place: the paperwork still has to be done but the admission can be expedited. However, there are other instances where a local inspector described in one case as 'a stickler' may not agree to fast-track such an approval and instead insist that the required paperwork is submitted in advance of admission. This may take some weeks, and by the time the approval has been granted the young person may have died. I was told of a number of such instances.

Once a TYA has been admitted, the difficulties are not over. In an interview with a participant, senior in the hospice movement, it became clear that provision for TYAs in adult hospices brings some challenges to both staff and patients. The TYAs were described as occupying a 'very uneasy mid-territory', not quite fitting anywhere. Although an adult hospice may care mainly for cancer patients (unlike a children's hospice), those patients will usually be much older people. As Liz said:

> Adult hospices absolutely do have the skills in terms of their disease process to care for them, but very often, if you talk to nurses in adult hospices, they will say, "I don't find it terribly easy to talk to teenagers – don't really know ... how to get to know them". It's not something that we do as a norm. That's a huge generalisation, but certainly from the young people's point of view, most of them will have been introduced to their local adult hospice and many of them will say to us, "They were really lovely and it was fine but I just didn't want to be in a ward surrounded by people in their seventies, eighties and nineties. I had nothing in common with them". So for them, very often, they will be the ones who say, "Actually, I don't want to go there". Even though the adult hospice might be saying "We could care for you", they may be saying, "Thanks very much, but actually that's not an environment I want to be in".
> (Liz)

Liz's comment is borne out by the story of Ellen, who died at 23 at home but who had been offered care at her local adult hospice. She was invited to visit with a view to her receiving her palliative care there. Her mother, Ann, told me this had been much too soon – about 3 years before her death, thus the timing was inappropriate. However, it may be difficult to calculate not only how soon death may occur but also at what point it is helpful for a young person to be familiarised with a potential care setting. In this case, however, the setting was clearly unacceptable to Ellen, and Sarah, who was involved in her care but not informed of this visit, said:

> She was deserted in the middle of a busy, adult ward and could see people who are really poorly. And I got a phone call from the Head of Care at the hospice to say, "Did you know that we've had one of your patients here today?" And I had no idea at all ... He said she sobbed ... She'd stood in the middle of the ward and sobbed and they went and rescued her, and she'd just been deserted. So she'd been taken into an inappropriate environment

and left ... it was terrible. And she did talk about it afterwards a little bit to
me ... I just think she found the whole experience a nightmare.
(Sarah)

The result of this unfortunate experience was that Ellen did not want to consider
the hospice as a possible care setting when end of life care later became
necessary. Despite this, at the end of her life Ellen received 'hospice at home'
care (discussed in Chapter 2). It is important to remember that although inpatient care at a hospice may not be age-appropriate, if the home environment
is suitable, home-based hospice services may be much more acceptable.

In Bianca's account of her visit with her young husband Ryan to an adult
hospice where he was offered end of life care, we see a similar response.
Although the facilities and environment were excellent and the staff friendly,
they felt out of place. For Ryan and Bianca the very term 'hospice' held dread;
to this young couple, a hospice was a place where people went to die. Although
Ryan had been told he would not survive, the concept was nevertheless
unacceptable to them. Bianca said:

I don't feel that they really understood us as a young couple. And in my
head a hospice was somewhere old people went to die and ... I was, like,
"There is no way you are going to be in this place". I was, like, "I don't care
how sick you are, you will stay at home and I will look after you", because ...
it felt safe at home and I really, really sort of fought for that. I was, like, "I'm
not letting him go". And even when people were, like, you know, his pain
needed to be managed ... we were both very much aware that going to the
hospice meant death, so I would say 3 days before he died, he was kind of
going in and out of consciousness and you could tell he was in a lot of pain
because when he was unconscious there was a lot of moaning, the nurse
was saying, "He needs to go to the hospice", and I [said], "No, he doesn't
want to be there. That to him means death, and if he's at home, he'll be
okay ...". It was full of older people and it was just somewhere that Ryan ...
shouldn't have had to have been. There was nothing there ... like it was lovely
and the rooms they showed us were really wonderful ... and the nurses were
really nice, but it was just ... no one was his age there. There was nothing that
I could relate to, and it did feel like this was somewhere people went to die.
(Bianca)

Bianca's interpretation of hospice care was that Ryan would be consigned
there to die and that keeping him out of the hospice meant keeping him 'safe',
despite his terminal diagnosis. In this case, although the facilities were
perceived as excellent, her phrase 'I don't feel that they really understood us
as a young couple' suggests that nothing would have encouraged Bianca and
Ryan to opt for hospice care.

We can see that the adult hospice environment is unappealing to a young
person, and that there are few services in adult hospices that focus on the
social difficulties experienced by the TYAs, such as employment, financial and

benefits problems. The staff were described by some participants as being 'rigid' about the TYAs' propensity to 'pad around in the early hours of the morning', and some staff found it difficult to manage their fierce, sometimes challenging, manifestations of independence and control, which can be swiftly followed by being needy, demanding and childlike. A balance also has to be struck between allowing the teenagers to 'be teenagers' and the needs of the older patients whose patterns, behaviours and preferences might be very different. Staff may also be unused to witnessing and supporting a patient who is 'dying out of time'. Young people can have very difficult deaths; paradoxically, although they are dying, their bodies are quite strong, 'they don't just gently fade away', and may be much more ill before they die, in contrast to an older person whose vital organs will not be as robust. Jenny, the Palliative and Supportive Care Tutor at an adult hospice, said that she and her team would know very little about how to care for a teenager. Although she said some training in advance would be useful to prepare staff for such care, she acknowledged that there would be little chance of interesting staff unless they were already faced with the care of someone in this age group – by which time it would be 'too late'. She suggested:

> To have sort of specialist centres that could be a Centre of Excellence … to be able to tap into … I would certainly be very happy to facilitate any education that needed to go out. But perhaps recommendations … [such as] five bullet points of things that could actually, you know, change … could actually happen in a positive way. I mean because the numbers are low doesn't mean to say it's any less important.
> (Jenny)

To tackle the anomalies and inconsistencies of admissions procedures for under-18s, some adult hospices have applied to have their licences extended to take younger patients, in the case of one adult hospice as young as 14. However, even regularising the provision of support for adolescents may not solve all the challenges. At one particular adult hospice, the implications for staff who had not chosen to work with teenagers were considered potentially problematic. Cherie, lead clinician at this hospice, said that over-16s having a boyfriend or girlfriend to stay overnight may be difficult for some staff. However, she said she would rather they were safe in the hospice than having sex in the car park. At the time of this interview, the consents were still being applied for and building work had not begun, but there were concerns about the design enabling the young people and the adults to be accommodated separately. Cherie summed up the challenges of this sensitive situation as follows:

> Well I think when I'm thinking of sort of teenagers and younger people, I'm sort of thinking sort of about all the risk-taking behaviours of that age group. You know, maybe sort of smoking some cannabis or wanting a girlfriend/boyfriend to sleep over and things like that – you know, have sexual relationships and stuff. And I think, you know, we just need to, you

know, highlight that these are the issues for these younger people – about peer group support. Also ... when they ... become independent as teenagers and [have] moved away, but then because of illnesses and circumstances they've maybe had to move home, and there may be, you know, relationship difficulties with parents, you know, and the dynamics that's caused from someone who's been independent, then becoming dependent on parents again ... The sort of younger people that I have worked with, there's been this drive actually to continue their education, even though, you know, prognosis is really quite poor, you know, they still want to sort of achieve something in the time that they have. So I think there's, you know, all these issues need to be highlighted to the psychosocial, or the whole team – the multidisciplinary team here ... When we've had patients here ... maybe they have gone in the garden and smoked some cannabis or something, you know, and it's like the anxieties that has raised in maybe some of the nurses that are here in the evening – you know, should they be allowing sort of 16/17/18-year-olds to go outside and do that or should they be telling their parents that they're doing that or ... you know, just the dilemmas it raises for people really. And I think if we're going to be lowering our age group, you know, we're going to come across more and more of things like that that we maybe need to sit and discuss as a team.
(Cherie)

Although drug-taking, drinking and sexual relationships would not occur in a paediatric environment or hospital setting, the issue may arise in an adult hospice and create dilemmas for staff, who may become caught between parents and their young adult children. It also raises the question of teenage visitors, how to establish what age they are and the need to ensure that illegal activity is not taking place on hospice premises. Sue B reflected on this:

Well, obviously we need to reiterate to people [parents] that people of 16 can have sexual relationships. But obviously because they are still under 18 you're going to have some very grey areas ... if people want to invite their mates round and have a drink in the room ... I can think of an occasion where we've had some under-18-year-olds drinking on the premises, you know, because they've done what teenagers do – brought in their cans and their alcopops and had a takeaway, and we've not known who's 16 and who's not. And are we then responsible for those people in our premises at night? Should they be ... under the influence of alcohol and then are we looking out and watching out for them too? So sometimes it's been a situation where we ... you know, the staff have felt almost like the babysitters, the childminders. It would create more issues if someone was under 16, because those issues about sexual activity and relationships would come into it. And lots of 15-year-olds, coming up 16, have got relationships. And if they're dying, and that's imminent, who are we to judge ...? I mean, there's a law there and we would have to abide by the law. But you know if you had a 15-years and 9-month-old girl who had been sleeping with her

> 16-year-old partner for the past year and she wanted to spend the night
> with him, I would have no problem as an individual saying that's absolutely
> fine by me, you know. But you would then have to consider the law and
> your duty of care to protect that person.
> (Sue B)

Other problems can arise when an adult hospice extends its provision to
teenagers, in learning how to facilitate the families who accompany them.
Sue B told me that younger siblings can sometimes be boisterous and need
amusing and 'containing', so they do not disturb the older patients. Although
she said that staff would be happy to undertake such care, they do not usually
have the time to do this. A 'sitter' may be used, but as Sue B said: 'Although
we are all CRB [Criminal Records Bureau] checked, lots of people have
different views and different values and they can often be projected'.
Nevertheless, Sue believed it was better for adult hospices to lower their age
range than for paediatric hospices to raise theirs, as she thought those
working in the paediatric environment might have developed a 'paternalistic'
approach, which would be difficult to change.

Sue was one of the few participants who mentioned the resistance young
people, newly sexually mature and aware, might have to being touched and
having their privacy 'violated'. She said that this might extend to therapies
such as massage in a way that would be unusual for an older patient who
would welcome such therapy:

> They're still very self-conscious and very aware if they've got a spot on
> their nose or they've got hairy legs, or ... I mean bodies are bodies to us.
> You know we're respectful but it's everybody's body and we respect
> everyone as individuals. But I think you have to have that acute awareness
> of teenagers [who] have to fit in with an image, and if they're not quite in
> that image, you know ... We have a hairdresser here, and we have someone
> that does massage, and someone that does your nails. But young people
> sometimes don't even like to be touched; you know they don't even like
> those touch therapies. "Oh, I couldn't have anybody massage me" ... what
> does that mean? Because we teach children not to let people in and touch
> you or handle you ... and lots of the therapies that we do are touch-
> orientated ... Older people who may be disfigured or lonely would thoroughly
> enjoy and embrace the human contact and the touch. But younger people
> might not be quite ... "It's a bit weird isn't it? Why would she want to come
> and do that to me", you know. And then we come, "Would you like an
> aromatherapy", "What's that funny old smell?" you know, "Oh that's a bit
> odd!". You know, you just don't know what's going to be acceptable to that
> person, whereas they might think it's far more acceptable to put some
> really loud, banging music on and shout, you know ... A young person might
> want to be up all night, playing loud music, gaming and you know, we've
> got to balance that with the other group of people that we have to care for.
> (Sue B)

However, even if the particular demands and preferences of TYAs can be met and the age-appropriate approach can be offered with staff training, Rosemarie, the Senior Palliative Care Nurse Specialist at an adult hospice, said that although there were two new rooms at her hospice that had been 'fitted out specifically with young people in mind with environmental control from the bed ... so they can have stereos playing and game systems', these rooms had not been used as much as they had hoped. She suspected that this was because the 'whole ethos' was not focused on young adults, thus the hospice in general was not appealing even though the individual rooms may have been. This is reminiscent of what Elaine said about the dedicated adolescent room at the children's hospice, and sug-gests that the provision of a sound system and games consoles does not address the issue adequately. Rosemarie identified another challenge: for some young adults there was no opportunity for 'transition' between adult and paediatric hospice services:

> The fact is we see people who've been in treatment for years and years. And for some of our young people with malignancies this isn't their first time. They've grown up with a malignancy, had treatment, been in remis-sion or cure, and now they've got either a recurrence or a second malig-nancy. So, for some of them, they've been down this route before and they've been under the children's palliative care team – very different ethos – and it's a complete shock when they then come into adult ser-vices, and expecting to be sort of nurtured the way that the children's team do. Whereas in the hard facts of adult palliative care the numbers are so great, and the resources, as few as they are ... it means that the sort of service cannot be the same as the children's service. So they don't have the transition because they're actually well during that period of sort of growing up, but they come into a very different service ... The youngest person I nursed about 10 years ago ... was in her early twenties and had had a very aggressive cancer. She'd had horrendous treatment. And we had to nurse her in a side room, which ... you know, we isolated her. Not meaning to. You know, with the best will in the world ... to give her that privacy and not mix her in with the older population that we had at the time. But, sort of looking back, with the experience I have now, I think that wasn't the best thing for her. You know that probably wasn't the best unit. It was the only unit available and her choices were very limited – it was either that or home. But her parents couldn't have cared for her at home, so it was that or hospital really.
> (Rosemarie)

Although it might be assumed that many young people have a boyfriend or girlfriend of their own age, one adult hospice had a difficult situation to manage with a young man of 20 whose partner was his mother's age. This resulted in the need for delicate negotiations, and some staff members found the situation problematic. Sue B told me the following:

> I can recall a young lad, a couple of Christmases ago, who was just early 20s - very early 20s - and how difficult that was for all of the staff. He had commenced a relationship with an older lady - a lady in her late 40s - and obviously his mum was of a similar age. And that was difficult for us all, because obviously the mum wanted to care for her child, and yet his lover/partner was of a similar age to his parent. And that was difficult for us all ... obviously we respected his rights. If that's what he wanted, he was over 18. But you know, your heart, as a mum, went out to the mum, you know. So I think there's lots of ladies of 40-plus here, and I think lots of people identified emotionally with that scenario ... in this young man's case, his partner was not his named next of kin, it was his mother. So obviously the partner then felt sort of out on a limb. But I don't think he really understood the consequences of not naming her. But I think it worked well, you know we worked between the two of them. They had their own time. We sort of allowed them to have a rota. But I think the partner did feel a little bit on the outside, because the mum was quite a jolly, overpowering character, who worked in theatre, and that was her nature anyhow, so I think it would have been difficult ... and he was her only child [and she was a single parent] ... So it must be very hard for the parent. And yes it does raise issues for us, but it's not for us to judge or comment on that, if that person's 16-plus and has made their decision, we can only respect their dignity and their privacy.
> (Sue B)

Sue B also told me that as this young man's life was drawing to an end, he wanted to have a last meal with his partner, and although this may have hastened the end of his life he was supported in his wish:

> He had an obstruction in his gut but had decided that he wanted to have his last supper. And it really was his last supper because he had a romantic meal with his partner, and enjoyed the meal and the wine, but within 2 hours he had perforated his gut and was in an awful lot of pain with that ... I think he fully understood [the risks]. You know his language was very colourful and explicit, you know. And some of the terms he used, you know, were blunt and to the point, but you had to come to his level to speak ... But that's a skill of every nurse, to arrive at the language level and the understanding of each patient and knowing how to pitch that.
> (Sue B)

Sue raises the important point here that all patients are accompanied by particular needs and demands and that staff have to be flexible and adaptive, but the examples here suggest that the needs and demands of young adults can be particularly taxing.

Despite the difficulties for both staff and young people documented above, there are examples of where adult hospice care for the age group has been flexible enough to encompass and meet the needs of the TYAs. As we have seen, paediatric and adult hospice provision can be unattractive to TYAs with cancer, which may account for why I have few examples of care in these settings. However, instances of how age-appropriate care can be delivered in an adult hospice setting are shown through the stories of both Simon and Sianne, which are now offered as exemplars of good practice.

Simon's story

Simon, an Australian aged 19 died from cancer in an adult hospice in London during his first and only overseas visit. Having been diagnosed with terminal cancer, he decided that having never previously left Australia he would spend the remainder of his life travelling with two of his friends, Peter and Tyson. The adult hospice in London where Simon received support allowed him to treat it like a 'hotel'. His needs became greater as his life drew to an end and his dependence on the hospice increased. After Simon's death, his mother, Helen, spoke of the sensitivity with which the staff had laid him out, respecting his youth culture. The age-appropriate nature of the care can best be summed up by his mother:

> They'd dressed him in his favourite black T-shirt and jeans. It was hard to get used to the dyed hair he'd had done just before he left. It was his last chance for a bit of teenage rebellion – black dye with purple highlights. (It sounds worse than it looked). The nurses said the purple came off on their hands.
> (Helen)

I include the lengthy quote from Helen below as I believe it shows that age-appropriate end of life care can be offered if the issues the young people are managing are understood and accommodated. Simon was not only a dying teenager, he was a dying teenager separated from his family and in a strange country and culture, yet the support he received could not have been tailored better to fit his needs – indeed it also encompassed the needs of his friends Peter and Tyson:

> The hospice people helped us to arrange the funeral (the wonderful Sandra helping us all the way through, the lovely Paula bringing in endless trays of tea). We didn't see Tyson and Peter that day, but the nun in charge of the hospice told us how great they'd been. They'd taken over the room, she said, there were bags of crisps and magazines strewn around. The doctor who'd been on duty when Simon died talked to us about the last hours. He was so sensitive and kind. The chaplain of the hospice took the funeral with the help of the local Anglican vicar who we'd asked for. We had no particular wish for a special funeral, since it was so far from home and we were still struggling with shock. Yet it became special. We were urged to use the hospice chapel, a small,

beautiful centuries-old domed building with a side entrance off the corridor near Simon's room. Nurses came. I'd asked that they not bring flowers; I felt they'd done everything to care for him, and that was enough. But Nicola and Debbie brought roses, an apricot-coloured bunch with a hand-written note: 'A short time in our lives, forever in our hearts'. Tyson and Peter gave us a gift too, in joining the procession into the chapel behind Simon's coffin.

I have an enormous respect for the care he was given at the hospice. The nurses were loving, the doctor compassionate and caring. The receptionist/administrator was endlessly helpful and understanding – quite special. They allowed Simon to face the end courageously. I feel he was able to keep on joking with his friends almost to the last because he could tell the staff his fears (reading between the lines of his file). The staff and Tyson and Peter did what I would have liked to do – they accompanied Simon through his dying. Simon was wise in going to London. These people weren't his parents; they loved him and cared for him as if they were.

(Helen)

Sianne's story

Candy, whose daughter Sianne died at the age of 20 in an adult hospice, spoke of how the hospice had made special provision and allowances because of her age. They had been sensitive to her need for as much independence and freedom as she could manage physically and had been flexible in their approach. Yet, we can also see from Candy's account that the staff were profoundly affected by this death 'before time'. Candy uses the word 'here' when speaking of the hospice because she is now the librarian at the hospice, which is also where the interview took place.

The first contact really that she had was by phone from a support worker. And, as her illness progressed, those regular phone calls did very much to support. I mean obviously I don't know exactly what was discussed in them but I know, you know, how much help they were to her. I know there were a couple of times when nurses sort of left the room very hurriedly, and it was because they were upset. I could see that, and I don't know whether Sianne was aware of it, but because of that age ... [it's] more upsetting, because it's not where your end of life should be ... it's even more so with young people because they get very few actually in the hospice ... They kept her room sort of basically open for her and said she could be at home or she could come in, whatever she wanted ... which obviously they wouldn't do for [an older patient] ... you know, you're either a patient or you're not. But they did their utmost to support her. She wanted to be at home to begin with ... But then when she was very breathless and was frightened she actually wanted to come in to the hospice because she felt safe and secure here.

Over the last couple of months, you know, because she came here for different treatments ... and because the consultants were so supportive ... like I say, they managed to sort her out with all [the] drugs and everything else, so that she could actually go on holiday on a couple of weeks ... So I think she trusted them and that gave her more confidence, I think, in actually being here ... She had her own room here ... she could do virtually what she wanted to anyway. It was like a home from home and she had a room where the door just opened out onto a garden, so it was private, so like just having the door open and sitting there ... They were very good here, and she could come and go as, within reason, she wanted to, as long as she told them where she was going ... She went out with her boyfriend for a couple of hours for a pizza and, you know, things like that. So I have to say that they were very good, which obviously, in a hospital, she wouldn't have been able to [do], you know.

(Candy)

In the cases of both Simon and Sianne, an adult hospice made allowances for the age and life stage of these young people. In an environment of much older people they nevertheless succeeded in providing an acceptable atmosphere and a safe and secure setting from which, when they were well enough, the young people had the freedom to go out with their friends. Indeed Simon appears to have been encouraged to use the hospice almost as a hotel from which to undertake his dying wish to see something of the world with his friends. In these cases separate facilities or an adolescent wing were not what was required, rather it was a philosophy of care, sensitive to age-appropriate support needs. Significantly, Sianne died in 1998 and Simon died in 1996 – 12 and 14 years, respectively, before data for this book were collected – yet the exemplary care they received in adult settings has not become the norm across the sector in the intervening years. However, these examples show that if the issues and challenges are addressed and the young people's needs are understood, even without additional resources and new build, it is clear that a philosophy of care can be implemented that allows young people to be supported appropriately.

Adolescent and young adult hospices

Understanding the reluctance of young adults to accept the children's care setting, and their unease at being placed in an adult setting with much older people, some hospices have gone beyond the provision of an adolescent room and have built an adolescent annexe for young adults up to 35/40 years old.

There are also a limited number of dedicated adolescent/young adult hospices such as Douglas House in Oxford and Martin House near Leeds where Whitby Lodge was set up for this age group. As Liz from Douglas House said:

> There was a growing population of young adults, who were living into young adulthood who previously would have died in childhood ... More of these children were living into their young adult lives and there was nowhere that would give them the support that children's hospices had been giving them in terms of access to routine respite.
> (Liz)

So we can see there was recognition that young adults needed a service that sat between paediatric and adult services, but that this was largely focused on young adults with complex life-limiting conditions rather than young adults with cancer. This age-specific hospice provision offers an ideal transition for the long-term users of children's hospices, bridging the gap between paediatric and adult services for young people with chronic life-limiting conditions. However, the excellent age-appropriate care setting provided by adolescent hospices may not necessarily be appealing to young adults with cancer seeking end of life care.

Douglas House was initially set up to support the children who had outgrown the environment of its sister hospice Helen House, which cares for children with complex life-limiting conditions. Liz explained that she had become increasingly aware that young adults with cancer needed such an age-appropriate hospice service, because when treatment was no longer an option they would be discharged home and 'basically it would be the families who would be caring for them'. Although they might have the support of a Macmillan nurse, there would still be a significant burden on the families who struggled – as described in the previous chapter.

However, extending services to young adults with cancer can be problematic for a number of different reasons: to the young adult with cancer, the profound physical and cognitive impairments of many of the service users can be challenging – as we saw with the paediatric hospice environment; and referrals may not be made on the assumption that cancer cases are not cared for in this setting and staff may not have the training in the appropriate skills set. To take these issues in turn: much work on supporting a young adult with cancer emphasises the importance to them of maintaining 'normality', which is key to the age group. However, they do not identify themselves with the young adult hospice users who, although close in age, are not familiar in any other way. If the young adult with cancer can be encouraged to give it a try, they can find it a supportive and reassuring environment, but they need to be willing to give it a chance. Mindful of these challenges, Sarah, the Director of Nursing at an adolescent hospice in the process of being established at the time of my interview, said of the challenge of providing care for adolescents with both cancer and non-cancer-related illness:

I think that's something that we need to think about for the hospice when it's built. You know, because that can be difficult when you have got young adults with cancer, and young adults with a non-cancer diagnosis. Certainly my experience, in my previous job, we ran a daycare service, and the young adults started to come into that daycare service. And we did mix young adults with cancer, and also there were boys with Duchenne [muscular dystrophy]. That worked very well. It didn't seem to cause any problems at all, and the young adults with cancer were very happy to talk to the young men where needed. And I think if it's approached carefully and sensitively it can work, but I think you have to think about the young people that you will have in the hospice. And that's obviously something that we will need to think about when the hospice is built.
(Sarah)

Similarly, Liz from Douglas House acknowledged the challenges but said that although the integration of the young adults with cancer had been an anxiety in advance, in the event it had proved not to be a major problem due to the skills of the staff who were very used to interacting with young adults. As she said:

Yes we did have concerns that maybe people with a sudden cancer diagnosis would find it difficult to be here with people with profound multiple learning disabilities who couldn't engage with them. But actually, in practice, it hasn't proved a problem. And I think that's because, even for a young adult who knows that they're dying from cancer, they actually still want to pack in as much living as they possibly can. They don't want to focus on dying, although they may need to do that for periods of time. When they have done that, when they maybe have had a very difficult conversation, when they have faced their fear or whatever it is, they then want to focus on living again. And that is something that the staff here are excellent at doing. Because all of the young people who've come here want to live – want to pack in as much as they can. So the fact that there are ... the facilities are able to support that, so in terms of, you know ... we've got a Jacuzzi, we've got an art room, we've got a music room, you know there are physical facilities here to enable people to go and have a bit of fun in one of those rooms ... the staff are superb at recognising and seizing the moment. So we might have a young adult with cancer in who's had an absolutely rubbish morning, their pain has been awful, they've had a dreadful time, but finally, by two o'clock, we've got on top of the pain, they've had a bit of a sleep, they wake up and they're feeling brilliant and say, "Gosh, I really fancy going out. I want..to have an ice-cream at the ice-cream parlour or really fancy going out for a film, or something like that". The staff here are superb at being able to say, "Okay, we'll do it!". They'll get the mini-bus out, they'll get in and they'll go. And that sort of thing is what we're able to support, because we've got one-to-one care and because we've got staff who've got that mindset, who are able to just

seize that moment. So recently we had a young lady in, very end stage with a melanoma and, as always, very complex family dynamics and she had had a very difficult time with pain and, as I say, you know, she woke up and things were okay and she said, "[I'd] really love to have a Chinese meal – love to go out to a Chinese restaurant and have a meal now". And so that happened.
(Liz)

Sheila, Head of Care for a children's/adolescent hospice, told a very similar story, emphasising the importance of choice:

I think one of the difficulties for the teenagers, and for us to be attractive, is that if they're quite well, even though they're palliative care, they want to be off out with their mates and not change their peer group. And that can be quite difficult, which is why we were saying that sometimes the children that then have a disability or a mobility issue find it ... easier. I think when you first walk in you may see a lot of children with a lot of disabilities, and that can be quite difficult to sort of come to terms with. I think, for the young people that have used us, they've found it very good to use because we are very flexible. There isn't really a routine, there is that one-to-one care so they can really take charge of their condition, which again on a ward can be quite difficult – and even at home can be quite difficult.
(Sheila)

Liz also emphasised the importance of changing the perceptions of the local health services about what a young adult hospice offered in order to get any referrals, as there was an assumption that the hospice was a respite centre for young adults with learning disabilities. Changing that perception had been a difficult and slow process requiring a concerted effort with local consultants, clinical nurse specialists and Macmillan nurses. Having cared effectively for a young adult with cancer had been the basis of succeeding in raising their profile in this area, and referrals are subsequently more likely.

Sheila, in a role similar to Liz's at a different adolescent hospice, emphasised the importance of liaising with the PTC oncology services rather than 'taking over':

The oncology families ... often have very good relationships with the oncology departments, especially in [this] area, and especially if they've relapsed. They've built those relationships up for a number of years and they don't want to lose that relationship, and they don't want, you know, someone to take over. So it is important in working in partnership.
(Sheila)

To incorporate both cancer-related illness and other life-limiting conditions in a single care setting has implications for the training of staff. Although the staff are expert in supporting young adults, some of the more 'acute skills' such as managing intravenous therapy, intravenous antibiotics and blood transfusions are necessary. Liz pointed out that skills around very complex symptom control and pain management are essential as the cancers that the young adults experience can be very aggressive. Sarah, too, acknowledged that many professionals who work in a paediatric or adolescent hospice environment might be unfamiliar with chemotherapy regimes and other cancer treatments:

> There has to be the understanding of the particular type of tumour and how the tumour develops. All the oncology training and background … is important, because the staff has to have an understanding of the chemo, the radiotherapy, the treatments that the young people have been through or are going to go through, an understanding of the trial drugs now that are being used in these young adults. And I do think that is very important because, on the whole, young adults will choose to be treated probably right the way through almost to the very end of their lives, because one of the most important things to them is to maintain hope. They do not want to give up. They really want to try every drug that they can that will obviously enable them to have as long a life as possible. (Sarah)

Although the very term 'hospice' might be associated with the end of life, particularly when the illness in question is cancer, Sarah stressed the need to avoid such an impression:

> Palliative care is about supporting the young person and their family throughout their treatment, throughout their illness and enabling them to live as full a life as possible. And that's where, I think, the psychosocial comes in. So it's to enable them to continue with their education if that's what they're wanting to do. It's to enable them and to encourage them to look at job opportunities if that's what they're wanting to do, to encourage them to maintain relationships, sexual relationships, maintain their peer relationships, because they often feel very isolated. They feel isolated from their peers; sometimes their peers perhaps have gone off to university and they perhaps can't do that. And so I think it's really important that the hospice movement is not just seen as death and dying, and end of life, it's about supporting that young person to enable them to have that full life, right the way through to the end … I think young adults often know that they have got very much shorter life expectancies, and they want to pack as much living as they can into that short life. So that might be experimenting with alcohol, experimenting with drugs. It may be wanting that sexual relationship before they die. But I think that's really important that we support them in a protected, in a safe environment and enable them to have those experiences, because they are not going to live long lives to be able to do that. So it's different. And I think

that's where the mentality is very different to the adult hospices who do a superb job, they really do, but they mostly focus on end of life and symptom control. Yes, very good psychosocial support, but it is very different when you're caring for young adults.
(Sarah)

Similarly, Sheila said the perception of hospice tended to be equated with 'end of life care' and suggested that 'impression management' was still a large part of what was necessary to 'sell' the hospice as an acceptable option to young people and their parents:

I think, for the young people with the wide range of conditions, hospice has become much more common than when we first opened. I think that [end of life] would have definitely been the perception 20 odd years ago. I think a lot of families, maybe if you're in that circle where you have a child with a life-limiting condition, have heard of hospices and what they can do. I think maybe in the oncology, because quite a lot of the children survive and do well, it's maybe not as well known as to what hospices can offer, and maybe they feel that that is ... that you go there to die, and using the adult model, where it's more in the terminal phases. And I think it's also down to professionals in how they sell us – I think that sounds an awful word – but how they say what we can do.
(Sheila)

Despite the fact that the emphasis is very much on life rather than death, the young people will have the opportunity to spend the remainder of their life at the hospice if that is what they choose. This contrasts with other hospice provision that may be limited in its availability:

Booked respite can be a week's stay, but longer obviously if they come in for end of life care then they will stay with us until they die.
(Sarah)

However, choice and autonomy are also important in this age group. Liz spoke of the occasional necessity to take a risk in order not to damage the relationship with the young adult:

One of the young ladies with a brain tumour who we were able to support ... was absolutely adamant she didn't want to stay ... She wanted to be able to go home every night, so she came in on a regular basis for daycare. She was able to come and she was able to have a massage and use the art room and have a session in the music room, and maybe have a Jacuzzi and then go home at the end of the day. And when it got very close to the end of her life she was in for a daycare visit and I did sit and chat with her and her mum, because she was really getting to the point where she was no longer safely able to transfer. And I was quite keen that they just stayed for one night to enable the occupational therapist to get some new bit of equipment in so that she could safely go home. But that absolutely wasn't what she wanted to do. So sometimes it is about that being prepared to be involved in risk taking. You know really, common sense said she needs to stay here just for a night to be safe but absolutely supporting that young adult to be autonomous and make their own decisions. She didn't want to stay so you know it would have been really unhelpful if we'd insisted and it would actually have really damaged our relationship.

(Liz)

Much of the discussion in this chapter – and indeed in this book – has separated the younger age group with complex, multiple and life-limiting conditions from the young adults with cancer. However, the overlap between these two cohorts is too often overlooked: the young adults who have lived all their lives with life-limiting conditions who develop cancer in adolescence or young adulthood. It might be tempting to assume that as long-term users of the services they are well supported, but according to Liz this is not necessarily the case:

One group who are particularly interesting are the young adults with cancer who also have another underlying condition. So, for example, we had a young man with Down's syndrome who then developed terminal testicular cancer. So if you add in additional issues like that, they really are at the bottom of the heap in terms of anybody being prepared to offer support to them. The most difficult death we had was a young lady who had cerebral palsy and then, on top of that, developed a malignant melanoma. And she lived just a mile away from her local adult hospice, but the family were told "We can't cope with her" ... So for a young adult who has some aspect of either physical or learning disability, and then on top of that gets a cancer, I would say the picture is even bleaker.

(Liz)

There were similar findings from the TCT end of life care service evaluation in which a CLIC Sargent social worker said: 'We have a 20-year old with learning disabilities – like a 5 to 6-year old. She would be better in a children's hospice, but was only offered a hospice for the elderly'. However, although Liz felt the picture was even bleaker for a young person with cancer as a co-morbidity, I also spoke to a health professional from a different area of the UK who told me that although she felt children and young adults with complex life-limiting conditions tended to be offered a very poor service, if they were then diagnosed with cancer their care improved, as cancer services are renowned for their high standards. These contrasting comments suggest that provision can be patchy; it may be excellent in some areas, but can be less than satisfactory in others.

Advance care planning

Whatever the setting of the hospice care, be it paediatric, adult or young adult, the hospice staff need to discuss carefully with parents what they should do in an emergency; Liz from Douglas House explained the process of advance care planning:

> One of the things that we do as an organisation, both in Helen House and at Douglas House, is ... discuss with the families what their wishes are around end of life ... It's advance care planning ... So we always have that conversation, that if the child or the young adult is moving into death due to disease progression, what do you want us to do, what level of escalation do you want us to go to? If they have a cardiac or respiratory arrest do you want us to keep them comfortable, do you want us to give them oxygen, do you want us to call an ambulance? And we do that planning for all of the relevant scenarios. So, for a child or young person who has a lot of seizure activity, it will be recognised that a possible way that they will die will be with a seizure that cannot be brought under control. So you know, if that occurs, "What do you want us to do? Do you want us to do everything we can here or do you want us to send them to hospital? If they go to hospital do you want them to go to ITU [intensive treatment unit], do you want them to be ventilated?". So we do that very, very detailed advance planning with every single family who uses us. So there are those difficult but very detailed discussions from very, very early on in our relationship, with all the families.
>
> So I think all of them will have done some thinking around actually what is going to happen. Absolutely there are some for whom death comes really quite unexpectedly, and there are some who, you know, you're absolutely convinced are going to die and actually they "change their minds". I mean it's a very interesting thing, the disease trajectory for older people with cancer is relatively predictable: once they start on a steady decline, actually you know you can be fairly accurate in your idea of how long it will be before they die. But children with complex health needs and also young adults, their disease trajectory, instead of being a sort of a downward slope maybe with a bit of ... a few plateaus on the way, they can be like a zig-zag. And it's not uncommon for these families to be told, on a number of occasions, that their child is dying and they need to prepare themselves for the fact, and actually then the child recovers. And we had that experience just 8 weeks ago – a young man who we've known for 6/7 years, came in and we were all completely convinced that he was going to die within the next 48 hours. And he's now at home and he's looking better than he has for the last year.
> (Liz)

This account demonstrates how difficult it may be to anticipate the course of illness in children and young adults, and that advance care planning may take place a long time before death actually occurs, but because death may occur suddenly and unexpectedly such a discussion needs to take place so that decisions have been made. The extent to which the child or young person is or 'should' be included in this discussion tends to be a matter of judgement and sometimes of disagreement between professionals and parents; their inclusion will depend not only on their chronological age but also on their capacity, competence and cognitive abilities (this is addressed in greater depth in Chapter 5). However, the CHANGE publications for both the carers of people with learning disabilities and matching texts for the people with learning difficulties may be a good starting point for such a discussion (CHANGE 2010a and 2010b). Although not aimed specifically at children or young people, these books are nevertheless presented in a very accessible way and the version written for the person with learning difficulties has a section explaining very clearly what an 'Advance Care Plan' is, and is illustrated appropriately.

Discussion

The data presented in this chapter represent the experiences and needs of two very distinct groups: those of children and young people with complex and life-limiting conditions and their families, and TYAs with cancer. We have also considered the perspective of the providers of hospice care, particularly the challenge of caring for TYAs with cancer. The data drawn from the children and families with complex and life-limiting conditions shows that the problems they faced were not primarily about the most appropriate place of care – indeed for those families fortunate enough to live in relative proximity to a children's hospice the place of care might seem obvious, whereas for the TYAs with cancer an appropriate hospice setting was much harder to identify. Paradoxically, these two cohorts regard the provision of inpatient care very differently: for the parents of the children with life-limiting conditions it is a lifeline, whereas for the parents of the young people with cancer and the TYAs themselves, inpatient hospice care may represent a failure to achieve a home death.

The challenge is the capacity and resources of children's hospices, which are funded largely by charitable donations. However, high the quality of the service, their inpatient and daycare facilities may be limited and unable to meet the needs of their users. Indeed, it is precisely the high levels of satisfaction and reliance on hospice services that can result in families feeling unable to articulate unmet needs and criticisms, for fear of appearing ungrateful and a concern that voicing criticisms or complaints could damage good relationships with staff on whom they are reliant. Nevertheless, even without additional resources there are ways of empowering users through the use of parents' forums and support groups and a willingness to be flexible in offering provision that can respond to crises.

The evidence so far indicates that, even with excellent clinical facilities and the best of intentions, the various hospice environments present challenges to both staff and patients when caring for adolescents and young adults at the end of life. So what can be done to meet the needs of TYAs? Hospices for adolescents and young adults can meet the needs of young people with chronic life-limiting conditions, and although this model works well and may offer an acceptable environment to young people with acute terminal illness, they are expensive to develop and currently few and far between. The option of building specialist hospice units for young adults with cancer is not financially feasible, so appropriate provision for young people with both chronic and acute conditions needs to be based on current services.

A number of measures might be able to address the challenge. First, with good communication, shared care between hospitals and hospices could be mutually beneficial, enabling hospice staff to help with the delivery of end of life care in a hospital setting, and staff from the age-specific care centres to offer support and advice to hospice staff after they have discharged a patient to their care. For such shared care to work requires good relationships to be established in advance between the hospital and hospice so that boundary issues do not arise. One way of achieving this might be the development of training packages that can be implemented if and when a young person in the age group requires support and care at the end of life. The need for good communication was taken one step further by a Professional Nursing Lead who participated in the TCT end of life care service evaluation (Grinyer and Barbarachild 2011), who discussed the possibility of reciprocal training as follows: 'working with hospices on a training exchange, especially if we start using hospices - and it'd be an education for them!' (Grinyer and Barbarachild 2011: 20). If this was established as a mutual exchange, the resource implications could be minimal yet deliver significant benefit for both parties. However, there may be sensitivities relating to professional status, as Clare, the Director of Clinical Services at a children's hospice said about shared care:

> Doctors talk to doctors ... I know, I've seen it ... I think that's probably key in how we get good shared care. I think doctors in acute hospitals, who are very busy, have to have utmost confidence ... who they're handing to are competent ... since we've employed two more consultants, our relationship with the Acute Trust has improved enormously ... [but] sadly true ... if I ... with a nursing background, was to ring up and said I had somebody who I was concerned about neurologically ... [it would not] hold the same kind of wellie as ... the doctors.
> (Clare)

Perhaps the best way to approach end of life care for TYAs is to develop a philosophy of care that borrows from specialist adolescent care in the acute setting. This can be applied in children's and adult hospices where, if it is possible to get the philosophy right, the physical setting can usually be adapted. For those few adolescent hospices that already base their care on this philosophy, it is a question of finding ways to ensure that the care setting is appealing to young people with acute illness and that they are integrated with the core users.

Lessons for best practice

We have seen the challenges experienced by those providing care in paediatric hospices in meeting the needs of the families of children with life-limiting illnesses, and the difficulties of extending their services to young adults with cancer. Similarly, the adult hospices do not offer an appealing setting to TYAs and struggle with licensing issues; whereas the adolescent hospices offer an attractive option for the young adults with life-limiting conditions and a more acceptable environment for the TYAs with cancer, they are few and far between and unlikely to become an option for all those who might benefit. So perhaps the key message, whatever the hospice setting, is worth reiterating: 'it's really important that the hospice movement is not just seen as death and dying, and end of life, it's about supporting that young person to enable them to have that full life, right the way through to the end' (Sarah). The following points are suggestions for changing policy and improving practice:

- It is not always clear to long-term users of paediatric hospice care when it is appropriate to expect a non-routine inpatient admission. The criteria for emergencies could be made more explicit to parents.
- Although inpatient respite care for children with life-limiting conditions is highly valued, the demands on parents in order to access this care can present challenges, and some families may feel it is almost not worth the effort; measures could be taken to streamline admissions and offer greater assistance with transport and travel.
- Where there is a lack of choice in the timing of inpatient respite care, parents may feel disempowered. Although the availability of beds is likely to limit the options, allowing parents greater choice would be beneficial.
- The development of users groups and an electronic support forum such as Facebook could reduce isolation for families.
- Transitional care for the TYA age group needs attention in most hospice settings. Children's hospices could consider the needs of their TYA users, who may value separate socialising space away from younger children. More facilities to meet the needs of the maturing long-term user could also help to attract TYAs with acute illness at the end of their lives.
- Adult hospices could consider applying for approval to admit under-18s, so that when an approach is made there is no delay in the paperwork required by the CQC. This setting could also benefit from considering the provision of age-appropriate facilities.
- Adolescent hospices are already well equipped for age-appropriate care; however, the challenge to them is to appeal to the TYA with cancer or other acute life-threatening illness, so that the balance of inpatient care becomes more mixed than might currently be the case.
- Shared care and reciprocal training opportunities for hospital palliative care clinicians and hospice staff could be developed, if lines of communication are established in advance.

Chapter 4
Hospital-based Palliative and End of Life Care

According to McCallum, Byrne and Bruera (2000), studies of the terminal stage of children's illnesses in a hospital setting are limited. These authors suggest that one reason for the paucity of research in this area may be a reluctance to accept that no further curative treatment is possible, and as a consequence health care professionals may be unwilling to approach parents to participate in studies on their child's end of life care. Another reason may be that proportionately few child hospital patients die, their deaths are from a broad range of illnesses and they are scattered across the health care delivery system, making research difficult.

Although the majority of children in hospital do not die, of those who do, most will die in a hospital setting so it is important that we understand what their experience and that of their families is like. According to Price and McFarlane (2009), despite most families preferring a child's death to take place at home, the percentage who die in hospital is high at 74%. This, they suggest, may be the result of limited choices and restricted options for other services and places of death. Nevertheless, they acknowledge that a hospital death may be the choice of parents who cannot support a home death and who need the security and support offered by a hospital's team of professionals. They also claim that in some cases a child who might prefer to be cared for at home will forego this if they realise that their parents cannot cope with a home death; although Davis (2009) cites Feudtner et al. (2002), who notes that some adolescents, after having lived all their lives with a life-limiting condition, may even prefer the familiar hospital environment. However, it is worth remembering that a preference for the 'familiarity' of a hospital environment may only be because there had been insufficient home-based or hospice services to enable care to take place anywhere else.

Brook, Vickers and Barber (2006) say that of the deaths in hospital, around 60% are due to complex, chronic, life-limiting conditions, and children with these conditions are likely to have prolonged hospitalisation and ventilation prior to their death. In a slight variation to this distribution, Davis (2009) reports that the majority of end of life care will take place in hospital specialist cancer units, intensive care wards and sometimes in accident and emergency

Palliative and End of Life Care for Children and Young People: Home, Hospice and Hospital, First Edition. Anne Grinyer.

departments. However, there is a discrepancy between infants and older children in the amount of time spent in hospitals; as Feudtner, DiGuiseppe and Neff (2003) say, infants who died spent a substantial proportion of their lives in hospital, whereas children and adolescents who died from complex chronic conditions spent most of the final year of their lives outside of hospital.

The McCallum, Byrne and Bruera (2000) study sought to document the course of care provided to children in hospitals, the goal being to describe symptom assessment, communication and end of life care decision making. The conclusions of their study show that a high percentage (83%) died in an intensive care unit (ICU) setting, 78% were intubated and the majority were comatose, sedated or medically paralysed. The interpretation offered is that 'excessively invasive treatment is being offered to children who are dying' (421). In 88% of the cases in this study there was no indication that the parents would have preferred the death to take place at home, but the authors acknowledge that this might have been because of the intensity of care needed. Of those parents who would have preferred a home setting (all oncology cases), all had to return to hospital for symptom control, hospital death being the 'default' position when a home death becomes unmanageable.

Davis points out that hospitals are geared to support acute and curative treatment rather than palliative and end of life care. As a result, they may not be able to meet the needs of children and young people who require end of life care and support. Indeed, Davis claims that studies from a number of countries suggest that hospitals seldom provide what families need; parents' accounts paint a bleak picture of the environment - overcrowded, lacking privacy, noisy, poorly furnished and poorly equipped are just some of the criticisms. Brook, Vickers and Barber (2006) concur with this, suggesting that, although it is possible to provide effective end of life care, too often the standards are poor. Aggressive curative treatments may be pursued with no clear benefit and the process may deny the child more appropriate palliative care. These authors also claim that the families of children dying in hospital report uncaring, confusing or inadequate communication; they feel that they have no control at the end of their child's life and experience more guilt, anxiety and depression after the death than those parents whose children die at home or in a hospice.

Sadly, accounts of bad experiences seem to be common and are replicated by Contro et al.'s (2004) study of paediatric palliative care services in the USA in which families reported distress caused by the uncaring delivery of bad news and careless remarks made by staff. However, what this study also demonstrated was the difficulty for staff in caring for dying children - staff reported feeling inexperienced in communicating with parents about end of life issues and said that there was little support for those who treat dying children. Again, in no sense were the clinical aspects of the care questioned or criticised - rather it was the emotional aspects of the care that were found to need greater attention, with both families and staff needing more support.

The pursuit of aggressive treatments at the end of life is also documented by Wolfe et al. (2000: 326), who suggest that for children who die of cancer this can result in 'substantial suffering' during their last month of life as attempts to control their symptoms are often unsuccessful, evidencing a need for specialised palliative care for children dying of cancer. These authors also say that although high-quality end of life care is now a standard expectation, it is not yet known if the care of children with cancer meets this standard.

Although Drake, Frost and Collins (2003) concur that there is a high degree of symptom burden for dying children, they claim that this is significantly reduced in the intensive care setting despite 'the vigour of intervention'. Their study also indicated that an agreement to Do Not Resuscitate (DNR) increased in tandem with the goal of treatment moving from life-saving to palliative. They report the number of discussions with parents increasing during this palliative phase when hope of survival had been lost, but say that 58% of the discussions with parents took place on the last day of their child's life. This suggests a limited amount of forward planning for the death and may be associated with reluctance to address the issue (McCallum, Byrne and Bruera 2000).

Hinds et al. (2005) undertook a study to establish what the preferences were for children dying of cancer and how their decisions had been influenced, and noted that previous studies had focused on the perspectives of clinicians and parents rather than on the child's preferences at the end of life, whereas, although their study included clinicians and parents, it was the young patients who were the main focus. Their findings indicate that the young participants – patients aged between 10 and 20 years – were aware of the gravity of the situation and not only understood the consequences of their decisions, but also showed an ability to enter into complex decision making, understanding the risk to themselves and to others. Hinds et al. argue that the young people (aged 10–20) demonstrated the characteristics of competent decision making, which is supporting evidence for the ability of young people to participate in the decision making process related to their end of life care. The factors considered of greatest importance by each group in Hinds et al.'s findings were: for the patients, avoiding adverse effects and having information from their health care professionals; for the parents, continuing to seek a cure or prolong life, trusting the staff, being supported by them and supporting their child's decision; for the professionals, the patient's prognosis and co-morbidities, and parent and family preferences. As with Contro et al.'s (2004) findings, Hinds et al. (2005) also found that clinicians believed that the assistance they could offer with end of life care decision making was inadequate.

After researching how the management of dying children could be improved, Ashby et al. (1991: 165) recommend a model that includes: privacy for family and friends; more sensitive body viewing, mortuary, autopsy and funeral arrangements; improved in-service education for staff, and improved information and psychosocial support for parents. They also propose the appointment of a specialist palliative care clinical nurse and consultant, the provision of specialised pain relief, and improved links with hospice palliative care teams, GPs and community nursing services. This paper was published in 1991 – 20 years before the data for this book were gathered; the question of whether this model has been adopted in any meaningful way in the intervening decades is addressed later in the chapter in the light of the empirical data.

Davis (2009) argues that children and their families need a room to themselves in order to ensure adequate space and a calm atmosphere. However, the likelihood of this being available to all children at the end of their lives does not seem very high. Davis also reminds us that even in a hospital setting the parents – usually the mother – will wish to continue as their child's main carer. The parents are the experts in their child's condition, particularly if it has been life-long, yet although they are experts in the care of their child, Davis says, they may be less familiar with what to expect at the end of life and need 'gentle preparation' (Davies 2009: 185) from health professionals. A quiet room where they can take 'time out' during this stressful period is to be welcomed, yet as Davis says this facility may be available rarely in a busy hospital where the only quiet place might be the hospital chapel.

In her US-based study, as early as 1977, Sourkes emphasised the many important ways that psychotherapists can support a dying child and their family. She noted the panic felt by some families even though death might not be imminent, whereas other families might be in denial of impending death when time was short. Thus, the therapist must be in tune with a family's rhythm. However, the danger of wanting to 'save' the dying child can also result in the therapist's over-involvement. Sourkes identifies four types of therapeutic intervention: the facilitation of communication both within the family and between the family and the professionals involved in the care of their child; the 'ongoing availability' of the therapist with the implicit understanding that the family can have an abiding trust in the therapist's availability; 'giving permission' to the parents to use the availability of the therapists to support their needs; and finally 'modelling skills' for the family thrown into crisis when suddenly faced with the hospital setting. Parents can feel like helpless onlookers and may lose confidence in their parenting skills, but care-giving skills modelled by the therapist can assist them to maintain or regain confidence, enabling them to regard themselves as part of the hospital team.

The recent development of a specific care pathway such as ACT's *Care Pathway to Support Extubation within a Children's Palliative Care Framework* (ACT 2011a) and its accompanying guide for parents in making critical care choices for their child at the end of life (ACT 2011b), may be used both to prepare for and support end of life care decisions. According to the launch material accompanying these resources, the pathway is designed as a flexible tool that can be adapted to fit with local policies; similarly the guide for parents (ACT 2011b) that complements the pathway is aimed at supporting families to make informed and realistic choices and covers issues such as:

- what critical care choices are
- what an end of life care plan is

- whether the child will continue to receive care and support and how symptom control continues to be of paramount importance
- the parents' continuing role in making choices about their child's critical care
- how critical care decisions are made.

The booklet also gives parents advice on how to talk to their child, how to communicate their preferences to the medical staff and agree a plan, and how to resolve disagreements between parents and doctors. Nevertheless, at the time of writing, these resources are very new and, although they may eventually act as a framework for both staff and parents to manage this difficult period and to guide decision making, currently the many variables that accompany the decisions made by both parents and medical staff regarding the death of a child, mean that the process 'has yet to be fully elucidated' (Drake, Frost and Collins 2003). It is the aim of this book to contribute to illuminating these processes through in-depth discussions with both parents and professionals who have been closely involved in the last days of a child's life.

This review of the literature on the death of children in hospital has focused on studies that address statistical information on where children die, and some more qualitative material on how children die and the impact on both their families and the staff caring for them. However, none of these studies addresses the changing needs of young people as they enter adolescence and young adulthood. Indeed, although the age range for the patients in Hinds et al.'s (2005) study was 10 to 20 years, there appeared to be no attempt to differentiate the changing and developing needs or abilities of the teenage and young adult age group in their sample. It is clear, however, that the young people in this age group, in transition from childhood to adulthood, have changing psychosocial needs and present different ethical and legal challenges for health professionals (e.g. Brannen et al. 1994; Apter 2001; Grinyer 2002a, 2007b).

Freyer (2004) addresses the issue of adolescence and end of life care, pointing out that for younger children the perception of death is less clear – it may be seen as temporary and reversible – whereas the adolescent will understand the concept not only in terms of its personal significance but also in terms of the impact it will have on others, primarily their family. This more accurate understanding of the meaning of death makes them a group distinctive from children, and the life-stage they have reached shapes their experience and impacts on those caring for them. Freyer describes the situation as 'a paradox of emerging capabilities and diminishing possibilities' (2004: 381).

According to Freyer, a number of legal and ethical issues make medical decision making problematic for the care of adolescents because of the issue of competency or capacity to make decisions. Adolescents may also disagree with their parents, who have up until relatively recently taken responsibility for decision making relating to treatment (Grinyer 2002a). Freyer (2004) points out that the legal status of end of life decision making by adolescents is evolving, may vary from state to state in the USA and differ between countries. Although it may be clear from a legal perspective in the UK[1] (ACT 2011c), the management of the situation can be challenging to both staff and parents. These legal issues of course also apply in the other settings of care addressed in the previous chapters; however, they are perhaps experienced most acutely in the hospital setting where decisions on moving from treatment to palliative care may first be faced.

Freyer (2004) maintains that excellent communication incorporating respect, candour and collaboration is the most important component of care for this age group. Clinicians should consider asking parents to leave the room during a physical examination if that is what the patient prefers. Such a request may be difficult for parents to hear, but if trust in the medical team has already been established, it will be respected as appropriate. The most difficult problem identified by Freyer is that posed by the situation where a parent refuses to allow the clinician to disclose the terminal prognosis to their adolescent son or daughter. He suggests that parents should be included in a commitment to truthfulness at an early stage, and that, if a parent continues to resist disclosure, the physician must make it clear that if asked directly they are obliged to tell the truth. This issue is discussed in further detail in the next chapter.

As with the examples in the preceding chapter on hospice-based care, an adolescent patient may find themselves in an inappropriate hospital care setting in a paediatric or adult ward (Grinyer 2007a). These issues are not addressed by Freyer (2004), although he does acknowledge that patients in this age group should not be expected to keep routine clinic appointments and that it is important to respect adolescents' need for modesty and privacy. He also recognises that upcoming life events such as trips, graduation and peer socialising are significant to the adolescent as are the sexual relationships older teenagers may have – these he says should be respected by the clinician. However, in paediatric or adult hospital settings such manifestations of adolescence may present challenges to staff unused to the age group.

The remainder of this chapter examines the hospital-based palliative and end of life care experienced by the families and young people from both the phases of the study: children with complex and life-limiting conditions and teenagers and young adults (TYAs) with cancer. There are also some

---

[1] In England, Wales and Northern Ireland, children over the age of 16 are presumed to be 'competent' to give informed consent or dissent to proposed medical treatments. According to the 'Fraser Guidelines', a child below the age of 16 may still be competent to give informed consent: '... whether or not a child is capable of giving the necessary consent will depend on the child's maturity and understanding and the nature of the consent required. The child must be capable of making a reasonable assessment of the advantages and disadvantages of the treatment proposed, so the consent, if given, can be properly and fairly described as true consent'. In Scottish Law, the age of presumed competence is 12 years. However, good medical practice includes parents in decision making under the age of 16 years. (ACT 2011c: 22).

accounts from health professionals, which illuminate the challenges to staff caring for a dying child. The limited material on hospitalisation from the families of children with life-limiting conditions is partly a function of the data on these children having been derived from an evaluation of children's hospice services, and partly because hospice- and home-based services were their main source of medical care and support. As we have seen from the literature, the majority of children who receive hospital care do not die, and those who do die in hospital are often not explicitly identified as being in receipt of 'end of life care', thus they are a difficult population to access through the hospital route. However, we may also learn about the experience of the children and their families if we approach them through their main setting of care – a hospice – as they are also a group that periodically uses hospital palliative care services. The data from the study of TYAs with cancer also illuminate issues relating both to cancer in this age group and to issues arising during end of life care for adolescents with other illnesses and conditions.

Findings

Concerns relating to hospital care

The focus of the interviews with the families of children with complex and life-limiting illnesses was primarily their evaluation of the hospice services used. However, they also talked about other sources of care and support, often in comparison to the hospice service, so it is possible to examine issues raised about hospital services. When hospital care was mentioned, experiences were usually comparatively negative in contrast to hospice care. Participants indicated that they would always prefer to draw on hospice support, and when they were uncertain of whether hospital or hospice was appropriate for their needs would rather call on the hospice first. This did not appear to be because the situation was likely to be more serious or life-threatening when hospital services were needed, but because they had developed a relationship of trust with the hospice and personal relationships with staff had been established in a way less likely to occur in a hospital setting.

Although the previous chapter indicates that some aspects of hospice care were experienced as less than ideal, it was nevertheless clear that participants had more confidence in their services. A number of reasons were given for reservations about hospital care; Susan, the mother of baby Barnie, for example, had concerns about the hospital where he was treated:

> When he has been poorly and in hospital, [the sister from the hospice] has always sorted him out; she has always been to the hospital to put his syringe drivers in. I prefer him to go to [the hospice] than the hospital, because there are not really any bugs as such. The hospital is so short-staffed.
> (Susan)

Although Susan acknowledged that the hospice too could be short-staffed, this did not cause her the same concern as the similar lack of staffing at the hospital. Susan's quote suggests she was also concerned about 'hospital bugs' in a way that did not concern her in relation to the hospice. Indeed, another participant in the service evaluation, Len, the foster father of a number of children with life-limiting conditions, spoke of one of his foster children as having died from a hospital acquired infection: '[He] had actually had an operation on his throat, and he picked up a hospital infection from there, and that is what we lost him with' (Len).

Lily told the story of her daughter Karen's birth in a military hospital, where it was suggested that a disabled child would jeopardise her [first] husband's career and the baby should not therefore be taken home:

> We nearly lost Karen when she was born ... she was born dead, "flat", and it took 20 minutes to resuscitate her. The military hospital couldn't cope, and told us not to keep her because it would affect my husband's prospects in the Army.
> (Lily)

Lily's account is culturally and historically situated, but betrays a particularly insensitive approach to the birth of a child with disabilities. Yet 21 years later, Lily's faith in the hospital where Karen had recently been treated was also limited. Karen received respite care from the local children's hospice while Lily and the rest of her family were abroad on holiday, but during her respite visit Karen became ill and had to be admitted to hospital. Lily was of course extremely concerned about Karen's welfare, but indicated that although she had been happy to leave Karen in the care of the hospice while she was away, she was not confident in the hospital care:

> She was actually hospitalised, so it was horrendous – but they [the hospice staff] were absolutely fantastic ... I got straight off the plane and went straight to [the] hospital and met there with one of the [hospice] outreach team, and she had been going daily to be with Karen ... I wasn't overly confident with the hospital, because they didn't know Karen.
> (Lily)

Both Lily and Susan said that it was the hospice staff who knew their children well so these were the staff in whom they placed their trust. This is partly a function of respite and outreach care from the hospice over a number of years ensuring familiarity with their children's conditions. However, in addition, the continuity of care and relationships built up with staff at a hospice reflect a comparatively personal service. In contrast, the staff turnover at a busy district general hospital (DGH) is likely to be much greater and relationships less personal, so the benefit of the hospice staff acting as 'advocates' for the child, whose condition and needs they understand, is important. Tania's son, Dan, died at home, but here she reflects on her unease at the prospect of a hospital death and what it would have entailed:

Two months before he died, we had managed to get his end of life plan in place. I don't think the hospital expected it to be quite as quick as it was – whereas [the hospice] tried to prepare us a lot better. In fact [the hospice] tried to prepare us for about 6 months before that eventuality, if I am honest. The hospital, our consultant, just had different views about ventilators and things that we didn't agree with. It all got a bit rocky at one point when what we wanted and what he [the consultant] felt was beneficial for Dan, it didn't agree ... We weren't going to put him on life support – we had made all of those decisions as a family. As a family afterwards, that has tortured us in some respects, me and my husband ... Did we have the right to do that, you know ... ? Who am I to decide that? I did it because I loved him and no other reason, but afterwards you question, "If I'd taken him to hospital, would he still be here?". So you question all of that. The truth of the matter is, he would have had a horrible, horrible death; the antibiotics needed for him would have accelerated his *C. difficile* so much he would have died terribly.
(Tania)

The differences in approach between the hospice and the hospital to Dan's impending death reflect Brook et al.'s (2006) suggestion of inappropriate, aggressive treatment being urged on reluctant families. This concern is echoed by Sue, a Teenage Cancer Trust (TCT) Programme Manager, who suggested that end of life care in a hospital setting could extend treatment beyond a point when it was productive or appropriate:

I think if the young person is in hospital ... medics tend to want to keep on treating, so they want to be proactive in their treatment and perhaps give more chemotherapy, more sessions of treatment [rather] than actually accepting that that patient is palliative and that their support and care needs to be set up in a different manner. So if they're under acute clinicians ... there's this thing, "Well, we're here to save people, you know, to prolong their life" ... even if they know that it's not actually going to happen ... I think there's a huge education issue of the medics, the clinicians.
(Sue)

While the data presented above on hospital care for the children with life-limiting conditions are not extensive, it nevertheless seems significant that these accounts of hospital experiences are negative or express some element of concern about what a hospital death would entail. Of course, the situations being discussed by the parents and families of children with complex and life-limiting conditions are in the context of a lifetime of engagement with both hospital and hospice services less familiar to the TYAs with cancer. Cancer diagnosed suddenly and unexpectedly in a young person, who has in the main previously enjoyed good health, means that the context of their palliative and end of life care is very different. It is to these issues that we now turn.

End of life care hospital settings for TYAs with cancer

As we saw in Chapter 1, the rank order of places where TYAs with cancer die is: hospital, home, hospice (Higginson and Thompson 2003; North West Cancer Intelligence Service 2010, see Chapter 1, Tables 1.2 and 1.3; NCIN 2011). Although hospitals may be the most usual place of death, the location may differ from the hospital where treatment has taken place. For example, the TYAs cared for on a TCT Unit, may find that their end of life care and death takes place in a different hospital setting. The TCT questionnaire responses (from a service evaluation I undertook in 2009) about the type of hospital environments patients died in outside the TCT setting, suggested that the young people died on a roughly equal mix of adult and paediatric wards, although one response replied 'never' to a death on a paediatric ward. The nine TCT service evaluation questionnaires – with one exception – reported very low numbers of deaths on the unit, mostly ones and twos. Of those units where the percentage of TCT unit deaths was calculated, they were estimated as follows:

- less than 20%
- less than 1%
- 10–20%
- approximately 40%
- two to three in the last year
- none so far.

The unit with most deaths (nine out of 70 patients referred each year) reported that of the nine young people who died four deaths took place on the unit, three out of choice but one young person became too ill to choose so the parents opted for the unit, and one young person died unexpectedly in an acute hospital ward out of the area (of the remaining four: three died at home and one at an adult hospice). Other hospital deaths recorded by units occurred in the paediatric or oncology wards of DGHs, but hospital deaths were reported as happening 'rarely through choice'. Indeed, one unit reported that 'young people die in hospital because no other options are available, i.e. at the weekend'.

The later TCT service evaluation of end of life care (Grinyer and Barbarachild 2011) generated the following data on hospital deaths for the year 2010 from seven participating TCT units of varying size:

- **Unit 1**: four patients died on the unit
- **Unit 2**: three patients died on the unit
- **Unit 3**: one patient died on the unit, one in A & E, three in hospital intensive care, one in hospital
- **Unit 4**: two patients died on the unit
- **Unit 5**: more than ten patients died on the unit
- **Unit 6**: four patients died on the unit
- **Unit 7**: one patient died on the unit.

Responses indicated that some of the hospital deaths were not the preference of the young people, who would have preferred to be at home, but lacking facilities in a community setting stayed in hospital.

It became apparent from this service evaluation (Grinyer and Barbarachild 2011) that there were different approaches to encouraging/allowing the TYAs to stay on the units to die – to some extent policy and practice was shaped by local conditions, resources and cultures. A nurse from Unit 2 said: 'If here is where someone wants to die, we should pull out all the stops' (Grinyer and Barbarachild 2011: 8). One unit indicated its flexible approach to accommodating a death because the young people know and trust the staff, are familiar and feel safe on the unit, as one staff nurse said: 'We do what's appropriate, rather than what's written down' (Grinyer and Barbarachild 2011: 8). However, these comments contrast starkly with a contribution from Unit 3 suggesting a reason why the number of deaths on that unit was so low; as the CLIC Sargent Social Worker from this Unit said: 'The Teenage Cancer Trust is about pain relief, preferred place of care, not about death.' (Grinyer and Barbarachild 2011: 8). It also became clear from another participant's response from Unit 3 that there were contradictory perceptions within the unit:

> We establish where a young person wants to be, and facilitate that ... perhaps away from the hospital. Young people [may want to die here] because it's very friendly in a teenage unit, unlike on an adult ward, and they have rapport with staff.
> (Lead Nurse: Unit 3) (Grinyer and Barbarachild 2011: 8)

In contrast, it may be tempting to assume that most of the TYAs would prefer to die at home, even though the TCT units are where they feel safe. Yet individual circumstances make it crucial that the patient's voice is heard, as they may have reasons for their preference for where they die, which may conflict with their parents' wishes. As the Lead TCT Nurse from Unit 6 said:

> What the patient wants is the most important – and that can be very different from what the parents want. We have to tread carefully. We had a recent case of a young man who was frightened to die at home, because he had memories of his grandfather dying in the room his parents had prepared for him.
> (Lead TCT Nurse: Unit 6) (Grinyer and Barbarachild 2011: 9)

Although the TCT units are the settings of care where there is the most experience and expertise in caring for the age group and the condition, it must be acknowledged that these units are primarily places of treatment not of palliative and end of life care. However, the service evaluation indicates that because the young people have felt safe in the TCT unit they may want to return there for their end of life care. As Ozzie, Professor of Adolescent Oncology, said:

> My feeling is that most of our teenagers and young adults don't get much choice in it. It's what's available. And they may say they want to go

in a hospice or not ... but I guess if you're in a unit, like a TYA unit like ours, because you've actually been so much part of that unit, and made welcome in that unit, I think that's the reason why a lot of people come back when they're in need.
(Ozzie)

Feeling safe and secure with the trusting relationships they have established in a TCT Unit, it is understandable that *in extremis* the young person and their family will want to seek end of life care in this environment. However, Ozzie also confirmed that although the security of end of life care in a TCT unit was desired by the patients, they may not have much choice: for example, a bed may be unavailable at the crucial time. However, Ozzie also said that there were those who showed 'amazing altruism' and relinquished the chance of dying on the ward because they knew how distressing it would be to the other patients. Indeed, I witnessed such an effect myself during a previous phase of the research: arriving on a TCT unit to undertake interviews, I experienced an uncharacteristic, but palpable, pall of gloom for which I could not account. The following day I was told it was the result of the distress felt by both the patients and staff at the unexpected death 2 days earlier of a young man during treatment.

Acknowledging that the TCT units are primarily places of treatment rather than end of life care, Vikky, a Nurse Consultant on a TCT unit, nevertheless said:

> We don't discourage people ... I think we'd have to have a huge change of philosophy if we didn't allow people to die on our unit. So therefore it is a place from diagnosis through to death if that's what's needed. I think the more troubling thing is where the young people should be ... That's the question that needs addressing ... for a young person on treatment for cancer, to encounter possibly eight, nine deaths within their treatment trajectory, I think, is very difficult ... I'm not saying that you should hide death, if anything I think sometimes if you manage it well and you demonstrate to another young person how a patient is being cared for and what you have available, I think it can be quite liberating for them, because they can see that other people have gone through it.
> (Vikky)

Although Vikky acknowledged that witnessing a number of deaths on a TCT unit can be distressing, she also suggested it might in some ways reassure other young people if it is managed well. This was not, however, Stuart's experience. Joan, whose son Stuart died in a DGH, told me how distressed he had been when a fellow patient died on the TCT unit where he was being treated:

> He'd seen other people die on him in there ... in the course of his long treatment and going in and out and stuff, I don't know whether he wanted to be another ... Two people died on the ward when he was around, and he just said to me, "Mum, oh God, that's awful".
> (Joan)

There is a limited number of TCT units in the UK, so, unless the patient's family happens to live nearby, the young person could be facing the end of their life far from home, and their friends may find it difficult to visit. Thus, it may not be the young person's preference, even though it is where they feel secure. However, Bianca's husband Ryan (aged 21), who was treated for 4 years on a TCT unit before his condition became terminal, was not offered the opportunity to die on the unit. Despite the philosophy of it being a place of care until death if necessary, the reality is that bed numbers are limited and as Bianca said:

> The Teenage Cancer Trust unit was just for when you were having treatment: it wasn't a place to go and die, because ... the unit ... want people to kind of have the best care whilst they're on there, so having people die but having that planned death managed ... wasn't what they did.
> (Bianca)

However, the alternative of dying in hospital on an adult ward was unacceptable to Bianca and Ryan because of Ryan's prior experience of such a care setting. As Bianca said:

> It was full of old people who would kind of moan about us talking loudly; about us playing music; about what we were watching in the day-room; there was nowhere that I could go and cook for Ryan ... I was only allowed to visit him at certain times. It was like walking on eggshells the whole time ... And it was a very difficult place to be together because they didn't want young people ... running around. Like we were active, we wanted to, you know, do stuff and spend time together, you know, playing computer games and ... just things like talking. People were, like, "Can you be quiet, please?".
> (Bianca)

Bianca's account shows how young people can find themselves in an inappropriate hospital ward – clearly, at nearly 22, Ryan was too old for a paediatric ward yet he did not fit on an adult ward where the patients tend to be so much older, particularly in an oncology setting. Nevertheless, wanting to receive end of life care at their local hospital was the preference of some young people. Wanting to be near home but not 'at home' may be connected with anxiety about pain control and parents' ability to cope with a home death. Sarah, a very experienced professional, said the following based on her observations of the decision making processes of young people:

> One of the things that they do worry about and they are concerned about is, will they have pain? "Will you be able to control my pain? Will you be able to look after me at home?" And also they're often very concerned about their parents – they don't want to see their parents upset. And they'll often choose to go back into hospital if they don't feel their parents

> are going to cope with them being at home. Because at the moment I think hospital is the environment where they feel safe. And I think if they feel that it's going to be hard for the family, they will almost make that decision to take that pressure off them and go back into hospital, because it's a safe environment: there's nurses available 24 hours, they know that they can access the pain relief if they need it. But ... they are worried: "Will I have pain, will you be able to control my symptoms?".
> (Sarah)

Yet Sarah also said she believed that when young adults are admitted to a hospital ward – perhaps for pain relief – it is often the belief of the consultant, the medical staff or the nursing staff, that they are too ill to go home, and that option is not explored, so they may instead become caught up in hospital politics and find it difficult to get discharged. She also thought that the paediatric care setting could display a reluctance to allow their patients to 'move on'. The young people are often well known to the consultants and nursing staff, and when they reach 18 or 19 they may not be transitioned into adult services because they are regarded as 'belonging to' to the paediatric services and are thus kept inappropriately in that service.

Shared care

Some young people who have been treated on a TCT unit but received end of life care in a DGH, may find themselves nearer home and 'safe' in a hospital, but the situation can be complex. Throughout the research, I heard from parents and professionals of incidents where shared care arrangements between the TCT/primary treatment centre (PTC) and the DGH became prob-lematic because of 'boundary disputes'. For example, Sarah said the following:

> The local consultants do not want to share care, so there's no provision made for them [the young people] for hospital admissions. So often they can be neutropenic, they can be extremely poorly, they can be febrile, and they have to go and sit in busy A & E departments and just be admitted to whichever ward is taking them for that day, whichever consultant happens to be taking them. Nobody knows about that young adult. Okay, they can correspond with the specialist hospitals, but there's no provision made at all for local shared care. And that has happened quite recently with a young man I was caring for. There wasn't a bed available in his specialist hospital; he went into his local hospital where he then died. Because what happens is, there is nobody really in the local hospital that knows that young person. It's frightening to go into your local hospital.
> (Sarah)

This quote from Sarah contrasts sharply with her earlier comments, in which she explains how the hospital environment may appeal to the young person because they believe it is where they will be kept 'safe' and pain-free. Indeed, it may be that TYAs' hopes for hospital care are not matched by the reality, and that shared care can present significant difficulties. I interviewed a number of bereaved families whose son or daughter had opted for a shared care arrangement and was told about professional jealousies between the PTC and the DGH in which the care of the young adult became entangled. I have selected some examples to illustrate the problems that can affect shared care arrangements.

Billie's story

Beckie's daughter, Billie aged 14, died at home, but received much of her palliative care in a DGH paediatric ward. Beckie had severe reservations about the quality of care in this setting and believed there was little understanding of Billie's susceptibility to infection:

> [There were] kids with all kinds of nasty [infections] ... they had measles and chickenpox, and ... [Billie] very rarely came out of neutropenia. And it was dirty as well ... it was dirty ... The cleaners would come in with their mops that they'd used in other [wards] ... you know, I was just fighting all the time ... I didn't feel comfortable doing that. I hate doing that; I'm not leery but I was proper leery when I was in there and I hated it. I couldn't sleep, because you never knew what was going to happen next. And there's occasions I just phoned them [at the TCT unit] and just said please get [us] out of here, they're going to kill her. I know why they do it, it's so you don't have to keep coming to the centre, because people live miles away. So you firstly go to your local hospital when they get infections or when they need certain chemos and stuff like that. And that's where the bulk of your care is supposed to be. But I don't know anybody that liked their shared care hospital; and not because they're rubbish hospitals ... they're just not ... specialist hospitals. So you go in and ... you know they'll try and put you on the ward – she can't go on the ward, she needs a cubicle ... they just don't know the routine ... they just don't know how to work with children – sick, sick children. Because the sick children they get are acute ... And I know more about her care than they do ... I mean because she was epileptic as well from the chemo, and you know it was just ... it was so stressful. And she developed allergies to everything. It was awful – horrible. And that's why – it's because they're not specialists. It's not because they're horrible people or whatever, but ... they don't understand that you spend half your life in a hospital ... so no, it's not okay for me to sleep on a chair because they can't find me a bed, and it's not okay for me not to be able to change her bedding and stuff like ... you know. Because I think in any shared care hospital – and I've heard it time and time again – they just don't ... they don't know. It's not the same. They're not a specialist hospital. With children, you know, you take your kids there; it's a battle to get anything. You've got people who don't know anything about oncology; they know nothing about oncology.
>
> (Beckie)

Although Becky's quote relates only to the hospital where Billie was treated, she indicates that among others she knows in the same position - and there were a number as she belonged to the bereavement group (see next chapter) - the other parents had very similar experiences and concerns. As she kept repeating, the fundamental problem lay in the fact that they were not specialist centres and did not have the necessary skills or expertise to care for a child at the end of life when dying from cancer.

Stuart's story

In contrast, Stuart's mother, Joan, described the shared care arrangements, between the TCT unit where Stuart had been cared for and the local DGH, as working well when he was under 18. However, Stuart was resistant to being in a paediatric ward where Joan said he used to be treated like 'a baby'. Joan reflected on how inappropriate the setting could feel, when her son Stuart died in hospital just before his 18th birthday:

> You know you're sitting there and you've got, like Dumbo on the wall, or you know, Goofy or Mickey Mouse or something ... and in the next room there's a baby of 6 months. And there was just nothing for him. You know, they come in and say, "We've got videos" - and they would all be, like, kid's stuff ... And you know, being bald and everything - it's obvious what's wrong with you when you've got a bald head or you look very skinny. That was always hard, especially when you're in there and people have just got the broken leg. Maybe if ... probably to go into a cancer unit that had a facility, it'd [have] been an easier environment than going into a general ward. But you know there's other people that are just there for minor things.
>
> (Joan)

Although he and his family had a high regard for the consultant, they nevertheless had reservations about other aspects of his care that suggest some similarities to Beckie's account:

> I was lucky that we had a consultant locally that ... who was brilliant ... I just used to phone her on her mobile when he was ill at home. And she'd get it all ready at the hospital for me. So she was really good. But yes, you do ... when you're actually in there, I mean I had to sort of be his frontline defence, because people would come and not know how to use a Hickman line ... I'd say to them that he's neutropenic, you cannot just ... anybody walk in and out, this doesn't happen.
>
> (Joan)

However, Joan became more concerned about Stuart's treatment as he approached the age of 18 and said that despite the care being offered in the same DGH, everything changed when he made the transition to adult care. As she said:

> Oh yes, they would just put him in an adult ward, and you're not allowed to stay. You know you get thrown out basically. They don't want you there ... What was the most annoying thing I found is, that they will not ... the local hospital doctors will not ring [the TCT unit] ... They will not ring a consultant. And they want you to go over the whole history again, as if they're going to come up with a different conclusion. You know, and I used to say to them, "Look this is pointless, it's wasting your time, it's wasting my time." Even with a shared care package, where you've got it all written down, I mean every time he went in hospital it was all written down what had happened. There was all his blood results; I mean they had everything there. They just couldn't be bothered to read it. Say well no, "Well you know - you tell us". And I'd say, "I don't want to go over it again". You know especially when you ... and Stuart used to say, like, "God where do you want to start?" ... I think there's a lot of this... you know, "Why do we need to ask them, we're doctors as well" ... There was a doctor on at the unit that the local [hospital] ... that had had been to TCT in London, so she was pretty on the ball and just said, "Oh no, we speak to London" ... But ... and the worst thing was, it was always late at night, you know, you'd get an idiot and you'd think, "Oh no ..." And they'd wait hours, and you're saying, "Look, he needs his blood now; just give him a blood transfusion".
>
> (Joan)

Joan told me she had tried to have Stuart readmitted to the TCT unit, but 'There was never a bed'. She also said how difficult it was to get him from their home in Kent to the London unit when he was very ill and neutropenic, leaving them most of the time with little option but to access local services.

Other young people were also faced with difficulties in their hospital care. Ann's daughter, Ellen, had a distressing experience on an adult ward that raises additional problematic issues, as Anne said:

> On a couple of occasions she was admitted as an emergency patient to the local hospital ... The emergency care there was fine, but once the emergency had passed she was sort of on a normal ward waiting ... In the bed next door there was an elderly patient and I believe he'd had a heart attack ... And the nurse came in and said to him that she needed to talk to him, just in case he had another heart attack. And he was obviously quite deaf, so this was in a very loud voice, and basically saying to him that, you

know, if he had another heart attack should they ... [resuscitate him] ...?
I was sort of like sitting there thinking, "Please don't have this conversation next to my daughter".
(Ann)

At 23, Ellen was on an appropriate ward in terms of her age, but as with Ryan's experience it felt inappropriate. It was also a mixed ward, and although Ann acknowledged that the elderly man's care was just as important as Ellen's, she nevertheless felt the care setting made the experience unnecessarily distressing for Ellen. Ellen in fact died at home, but after Chris's son, Ben, left the care of a TCT unit, he died on an adult ward after having been previously treated on a paediatric ward during his experience of shared care. Chris's account is remarkably similar to Joan's, drawing the distinction between adult and pediatric DGH care settings:

> He started off at the paediatric unit at [the DGH] and they were fantastic – absolutely fantastic. But there was such a mixture of ages. I mean, he could have a baby of 2 months next to him, and it really wasn't right. He was 16/17 and there was youngsters running around, toddlers running around, so it really wasn't suitable. But, the care there was quite good. When he reached 18 we were told that he would probably have to go over to the adult services. I can remember going to look round the adult ward – the adult cancer ward – with Ben. It was just horror. I walked in and it was awful. It just wasn't set up for teenagers at all. I was absolutely devastated and I was crying. She [the doctor] took me out and I said, "I'm sorry, but you know ...". And I kept apologising to Ben, because Ben was with me too. And I obviously didn't want to worry him but I thought, "This isn't right for teenagers. He can't be next to an old, elderly gentleman using a commode with just a curtain pulled between them". There was nothing – there was nothing for teenagers. There was no nice TVs or anything to make their life comfortable. I mean, to be honest, we sort of looked at [the DGH] just as somewhere if we need to go desperate ... urgently ... Whenever he was ill, if ever he had a temperature we would take him straight to [the PTC]. We never, ever used [the DGH] until, strangely enough, his last few days we had to take him there. The palliative doctor said he needed treatment. He felt he had pneumonia. He'd rung the [the PTC] and they said it was better to go to the local hospital, and so we really had no choice ... We would have preferred him to have gone to the [the PTC] – it was what he was used to. He knew all the nurses, he knew the staff there. But, saying that, he was taken to [the DGH] and ended up in intensive care, who were absolutely fantastic and treated ... him for pneumonia. He was put into what they call induced coma, to try and let the drugs work and Ben knew they were treating him. Even though we knew he was terminal, he was told he was being treated. And he never did come out of the induced coma, but he went fighting ... and I don't think that

> would have been the case if he'd have gone to the [the PTC]. I think, because they knew him so well, and they knew that he ... there wasn't a cure, they knew that ... they knew how his body was working, I don't think he would have been treated. I think he would have been given maybe the option of coming home with a syringe driver.
>
> (Chris)

Although Clare's son, Joe, actually died at home, her experiences of arranging palliative shared care with the local DGH were equally problematic, because the DGH oncology services refused to take responsibility for any of Joe's care unless they took over his case in its entirety.

> There was a time when Joe had a problem when his bowels were blocked ... it was the chemotherapy had affected his bowel movement ... There was a couple of times when we needed care ... we did go to the hospital this one time ... because of this bowel, they said that he couldn't have shared care because he was under [the PTC] for all of his care, and unless they took over the whole of his care they wouldn't see him as a patient on their oncology side. So he would have to go through the normal emergency procedure of going through outpatients and ... or going through the emergency department and seeing triage, and then waiting for a doctor to come down, and then ended up on whatever ward he was put. And they wouldn't take him, unless they took over all of his care ... at that time he'd been under [the PTC] since the age of 15 so ... you know his care was there ... different hospitals, local hospitals ... all said the same thing, that they wouldn't take him unless they took over all of his care ... He had a week in [the DGH] with this constipation – nothing was sort of working – and he was very unwell. He ended up on a ward ... where they had a spare bed really. And the consultant of that ward, he wrote to the person that deals with the oncology there to say, you know, " I've got this young man, please will you see him. If this ever happens again, if he ever needs shared care, will you be prepared to say that, yes he can go in there and get it?". And they come back and said, "No".
> (Clare)

Commenting on the issues that can make shared care problematic, TCT Nurse Consultant Vikky made the following observations:

> Local paediatricians try very hard if they're a dedicated paediatric oncology shared care centre, to actually really work with us ... For the under-16 s, I think it's very well defined. But you still have that same issue that within the British Health Service it does seem to be that your 16–18-year-olds, whether you're needing to have IV antibiotics, whether you're needing end of life care, you seem to fall through. There is no

real ... provision. [If] you look at other things, like our National Service Framework, they talk about care going up to 18 ... But then you talk to local paediatricians who are told they can't take anybody over 16, and then your adult colleagues don't want to take anybody under 18. So, wherever you look within the health services, there is someone that falls through the gap.

(Vikky)

Interestingly, Vikky identifies a potential gap in services for the 16–18-year-olds in hospital care remarkably similar to the gap identified in community-based care discussed in Chapter 2. However, Vikky was at pains to point out the input of the excellent hospital-based palliative care teams who liaise well with local services and whose outreach work extends to local services. Nevertheless, she acknowledged that there is something of a 'postcode lottery', which results in some regions and localities receiving excellent support based on cooperation and goodwill whereas others fare less well: 'We have some wonderful shared consultants ... [but] you're dependent on individuals rather than it being uniform across the country' (Vikky).

As Liz said in Chapter 3, some children with life-limiting conditions develop cancer, likewise, some TYAs who develop cancer have other conditions – even if they are not life-limiting – which may affect their care needs. Amy, aged 13, who had Asperger's syndrome, had been treated on a TCT unit but her death took place on the intensive care ward of the same hospital. Amy's mother Pam told me about the events leading up to her death:

> Amy had Asperger's syndrome as well, and therefore you know some of her ways of thinking obviously were not like you and I, and so therefore things had to be adapted for her so that she could cope with things. And she was very much a black and white person ... And if we'd said the words to her, "You are not going to get better", I don't think she would have coped with that ... because she was always a very hopeful person and a very positive person ... [In the end] it was very unexpected and it was very quick ... These two nights prior [to her death] were very bad ... so bad that I had to call the nurse in on both occasions to try and help me calm her down. And the night before the Thursday morning, which was her last day, she actually woke up in the middle of the night in a terrible, terrible panic and she looked at me and she said, "I'm dead, aren't I?" ... and I said, "No, no, of course you're not". "Yes I am" she said, "I know I am". She said, "I know that I've all been mangled up and I've been put back together, but I'm dead" ... And you know it took myself and a nurse quite a little time to calm her down. And then the next morning, on the Thursday, her last day, she started being unable to breathe. And obviously the consultants all came in and they decided that she had to go down to intensive care. And so you know, obviously that was very

frightening for her because the unit had become a secure [place] and she was used to all her nurses there. And Amy liked familiarity, and so that was very scary for her, to be taken to intensive care, but we understood why she had to go.

And basically the day just went from bad to worse. And her breathing was so bad, and what they discovered was that all her lungs were filling with fluid … And so I was called into a meeting with the consultants - Nick [Amy's father] stayed with Amy. And they just basically said that the only choice they had really, was to give her an anaesthetic and put her to sleep so that her body could try and get through this, but they were 90% sure that she wouldn't wake up. So I had to give them the permission for them to give them the anaesthetic.

But before I went into the meeting with the consultants, Amy was begging, begging me to get the doctors to do something, because she was getting so distressed. Amy had always liked to have an anaesthetic, she called it a 'magic sleep', and she liked having a magic sleep. She'd never been frightened of them and she'd had … well it must be a hundred during all her treatment. So they said that she could have an anaesthetic and … they told me there was no chance that she would get over this … and so I said, "How soon is she going to have this magic sleep?" and they said, "Immediately, straight away, within the next 15 minutes". And I said, "I don't want Amy to know she's not going to wake up" … and they said, "No, I think that's understandable" … it was so hard. It was so hard to make that decision … Then I went back in with Amy, and Nick went in with the consultants, because obviously he had to be told too, and I couldn't tell him. So Nick went in, and fortunately he also agreed that was what had to be done. And when I went back in with Amy I just told her, very calmly, I said, "Rachael …" - that's her consultant who Amy loved - I said, "Rachael has decided the best thing Amy" I said, "is for you to have a magic sleep". I said, "And then when you wake up you'll feel a lot better". She said, "Oh, thank you!" "Thank you", she said, "for telling Rachael they can give me a magic sleep". And then Nick came back in, and the doctors all came back in, and they were just so lovely with her. And she just drifted off very calmly … she was so calm. There was no panic, nothing. And she drifted off to sleep. And that was it. And they really tried to save her. The doctors came in and they tried to do things to her. And they told us afterwards that she really put up a fight. But then she had a cardiac arrest. She died …

(Pam)

Although Amy did not die on the TCT unit where she had been treated, it seems there was continuity of care in the hospital. We hear that Amy's consultant 'who Amy loved' was a constant presence and reassuring under the circumstances for both Amy and her parents. Amy's Asperger's syndrome meant that she needed familiarity to feel safe, and although she had to be taken from the TCT unit to intensive care, at least it was in the same building and she was accompanied by staff who knew her well and in whom she had placed her trust. Had this crisis been managed by a DGH, it is likely that although the outcome would have been the same, the process would have been more distressing for Amy who simply looked forward to her 'magic sleep'; a term the TCT staff understood was significant and reassuring to her. This echoes the comments earlier in this chapter from both Susan and Karen, who spoke of the reassuring value of having hospice staff familiar with their children's conditions present at the hospital. However, although Amy's special needs were managed with sensitivity, this example raises issues of capacity and competence and how end of life decisions are made – particularly for a child under the age of consent who has some cognitive impairment. These themes will be examined in greater detail in the following chapter.

Case study: Nathan

To illustrate some of the issues that arise for professionals during the care of a young adult with cancer, I have selected the case study of a young man, Nathan, who died on the paediatric ward of a DGH at the age of 15. The example has been selected not because it demonstrates the potential pitfalls of such a situation described above by a number of parents, but because it shows that even in a setting where all those involved are committed to providing the best possible environment and support system, certain challenges appear inevitable under such circumstances. In this instance Nathan had the choice of being cared for in an alternative setting at his PTC, but chose his local paediatric facility as it was near to home, family and friends. There were no boundary disputes between the PTC and the DGH; indeed, it seems that there was considerable collaboration and cooperation between services, and real concern by staff underpinned the care Nathan was given and the support offered to his family. Nevertheless, a number of issues relating to the situation arose.

I first learned of Nathan's case during an interview with Alison, the lead cancer nurse in the oncology unit at the DGH in question. She had had no direct input into Nathan's care but told me that discussions with the line managers involved had alerted her to the fact that his care had raised a number of issues. Her concerns related both to Nathan's wellbeing and the welfare of the staff responsible for his care, who she believed were not well prepared to support either him or themselves; indeed, she said his case had caused some trauma to staff members. Referring to the expertise of the staff she said:

> We probably over-care for them in secondary care, because we haven't got the knowledge and skills to support them … We'll encompass them and become paternalistic with them maybe, and not allow them to be themselves and express themselves potentially, because we want to care for them so much, and we want to do everything for them and make this very traumatic experience as pain-free as we can.
> (Alison)

Alison also expressed considerable concern for the wellbeing of the staff caring for Nathan. Although the staff in question received clinical supervision, her concern was that they needed additional support in delivering care in what she described as very unusual circumstances. As she said:

> One or two of the staff have really struggled following this child's death. And they've become very attached to the parents, and that professional and personal relationship boundary has become muddied. And I'm not saying that that's wrong – but is that right and is that healthy for the health professional?
> (Alison)

One of the concerns expressed by Alison related to how Nathan's treatment was delivered. Because the staff on the paediatric ward did not have the expertise in administering chemotherapy, for a period of time Nathan underwent a 120-mile round trip each day by ambulance to the PTC for his chemotherapy, this left the pharmacist deeply concerned:

> Well, that was what was traumatising the pharmacist that contacted me about the patient, because he was aware that this chap was going down to [the PTC] every day, and then coming back to be fed overnight [here], and then going back and coming back ... It was only a short chemotherapy treatment, so the question the pharmacist asked me was, with my expertise of chemotherapy could we not deliver the chemotherapy locally, and then he could just stay in one place? But guidance is there – and this is where sometimes ... it's that fine line between what is clinically safe, taking governance into consideration, and what is right for an individual patient. And it's a really hard and fine line.
> (Alison)

At the age of nearly 16, Nathan would be among the older patients on the ward. When I visited this ward I could see the effort that had been made to make it an environment that would appeal to young children. Yet it was the place that Nathan chose to be treated. The alternative for Nathan would have been the PTC at the children's hospital 60 miles from his home, where he could have been admitted as an inpatient. Having realised that Nathan's case raised a number of important issues, I arranged to interview John and Wendy, both centrally involved in his care.

John is the ward manager for paediatric inpatient services at the DGH where Nathan was cared for and eventually died. John emphasised that the staff on the ward 'did a fantastic job' caring for Nathan, and that the ward had a shared care protocol with the PTC, which was put into operation for the first time in his case. The shared cared arrangement appeared to work well in the liaison between the ward and the PTC's oncology nurses, and on several occasions the outreach nurses from that centre visited the ward to offer help and guidance. John was aware of the age-specific TCT unit situated not far from the PTC but said, 'I don't know very much about those'. Thus, it seems there was no attempt by any of Nathan's carers to access expert advice from this source of potential support. Interestingly, John emphasised the challenge of caring for a teenager or adolescent regardless of their illness:

> I think there are big issues in a district general hospital about us not being able to provide appropriate care for any adolescent, irrespective of what their illness may be. I think that, because of the nature of what we do, we're sort of "Jacks of all trades". We have to be able to deal with anything that comes through the door, initially anyway. If it needs further help then it goes to a specialist centre. But there is a big gap in DGH provision for adolescents, particularly as we're talking about cancer patients – but also any other adolescent.
>
> We do not have the time, as an acute hospital setting, to spend with the teenagers that we would want ... we haven't got the staff, we haven't got the time to do it. And that's what I think actually frustrates staff in looking after these sorts of the teenagers, more than anything else, is they see a child in need, they see a child in pain – whether it be physical or whether it be psychological pain – and they want to be there for that child ... They come into nursing to nurse; they're empathetic, they're sympathetic and they want to do that. And at the end of the day, because we're so busy, we can't do that, we don't have the time. You know you want to come in and talk to a child who you know is dying, and they know is dying – and they want to talk about things. They want to talk about the trip that they've just been on ... they want to share those experiences. The family might not be around, or they want to talk to you about something that they daren't talk about to the family – you have not got the time to do that ... I mean in [Nathan's] case, night-time was the time when the staff did have a little bit more time and they would go and talk to him for a period of time. But, even then, you're always conscious, you go into the room, you talk to them, I've got a million and one other things that I've got to do. I can't give my full undivided attention to this individual because I'm always thinking that I've got to go in 10 minutes, 15 minutes, to do something else. That's the big, big frustration. (John)

John also talked about the difficult family dynamic that can occur when caring for a teenager – how much do you tell them? How much do they know? Are the parents trying to protect them by keeping them ignorant of their prognosis? Who has told what to whom? As a result of such confusion and uncertainty, communication can break down. Of course, the issue of sharing information with teenagers may be very difficult for staff to manage, when their expertise lies in caring for much younger children whose parents are likely to be the recipients of information and to be the decision makers.

Nathan was in a single room most of the time, primarily because of the risk of infection, and John told me that they had allowed Nathan to decorate it as he wanted with big sheets of paper on which they made football scenes. So the room was personalised but, as John said:

Not quite sure what the fire officer would have made of it if he'd seen it, but my attitude would be, "Well I'm sorry, tough! This kid has not got long to live ... you know we've got to make this as nice, as dignified and as pleasant an experience as we possibly can".
(John)

Wendy, the ward's clinical lead nurse, said many of the issues relating to oncology were new to the ward as most paediatric cancer cases are treated in a tertiary or specialist centre. However, Nathan had been under their care for much of his treatment for a period of 18 months, and, although there was shared care with the PTC, the paediatric ward took most of the responsibility. It was Nathan's choice that his care took place on the ward, apart from the chemotherapy and radiotherapy, which Wendy described as being 'out of our capabilities'. She pointed out how important it was that shared care worked, as parents cannot be expected to travel a 100-mile round trip with their sick son or daughter every time they need a blood test. However, she also said that their training needs were an issue, because of the importance of keeping knowledge up to date in the DGH so they can deal with the unexpected. She also acknowledged that although she and her colleagues accepted that 'we're just an assistant', in other hospitals there were professional jealousies and boundary issues that resulted in an attitude of 'they're our patients and we'll deal with them'. She said of Nathan's end of life care:

When it became apparent that his treatment wasn't going to be successful, then obviously to us that was very important as well. And it was kind of a privilege [for us] for him to say that he wanted to be here and be with us, because we became part of his family, really. But for us and for our staff, and for me particularly, that was very tough because ... if we see death it's very often ... children that come in through A & E suddenly, in road traffic accidents and things. But to live through something with somebody for 18 months and then not to have a positive outcome at the end of it, you know, we all found very difficult ... You know, we're not used to failing people because they come in ill, they get better, they go home.
(Wendy)

It was clear that Nathan's death had had an ongoing impact on Wendy and the other staff who had cared for him. She continued by telling me that after Nathan's death staff felt they needed support from counselling, describing their emotional resources as being drained. Unusually, Wendy said she still sees Nathan's mother regularly to support her and his mother also visits the ward where he died to see other staff who cared for him. Although Wendy indicated that she wished to support Nathan's mother, I had a sense that the emotional impact his death had had on her meant that she, too, found some solace in this ongoing contact; nevertheless, it is unusual for such a lasting bond to be formed with a parent.

Staff are, of course, also affected by their care of other chronically sick children, and Wendy said they need support, which is not necessarily being provided:

> The staff do need some kind of a support. You know we deal with quite a lot of children with cystic fibrosis who obviously ... have got long-term health needs. And some of them, you know, are really sick children. And it's very difficult to deal with them, to support them and their families day in, day out ... because you take on board their stresses and their emotions. And I think they do realise that you know there is, you know, a lapse in the service there, but I'm not sure whether anything's, you know, being done about it. (Wendy)

Despite the clear need for greater emotional support for staff caring for children with a range of conditions, I nevertheless had the sense that Nathan in particular had made a lasting impression on all who had cared for him. The impact his case and care had had on the staff, even a year after the event, was obvious. Indeed, the room where I undertook the interviews had been planned by him and named after him and was used as a counselling room at his request; he chose the colours, paintings and design, and lives on in a very palpable way in the life of the ward.

Discussion

Although there are relatively few accounts of hospital care from the families of children with life-limiting conditions, we can see that the data from them and from families of the TYAs with cancer confirm the concerns raised by the literature at the start of this chapter, and provide in-depth personal accounts that lend detail to the statistics. Both the parents of children with complex life-limiting conditions and those of young adults with cancer had similar reservations and concerns about the hospital environment. In contrast with either the hospice setting or the specialist cancer setting, there was a feeling that their child's end of life needs were not understood by staff in the general hospital ward. Whether this was a concern about infection, communication or an age-inappropriate environment, parents tended to feel hospital services were an option of last resort – in some cases to be avoided at all costs.

The reports of both parents and professionals indicate that shared care arrangements do not always result in the expertise of the PTC being welcomed in the DGH. Professional boundaries and the 'ownership' of the patient and their care appear to lead to a degree of unwillingness to share the case, with the patients and their families becoming caught up in inter-hospital politics. This reluctance to share care was confirmed by Sarah as not being related to accountability and the fear of 'blame' if the regime proved problematic, but because the DGH oncologists do not know the PTC consultants. This suggests that communications between the PTC and the DGH are crucial to shared care and need to be established early, well before a crisis occurs. Indeed, the one exception was related by Stuart's mother Joan who said: 'There was a doctor on at the unit that the local [hospital] ... that had been to TCT in London, so she was pretty on the ball and just said, "Oh no, we speak to London", thus indicating that where relationships have been established and visits made to specialist units by DHG staff this can overcome boundary issues and the reluctance to share care. These boundary issues and shared care problems may, however, be mitigated in the case of children with long-term life-limiting illness who appeared to continue to benefit from the input of hospice services even while in hospital. This may be because the esoteric needs of these children contrast with those of the cancer patients, of whose care the DGH oncologists wish to take ownership.

However, I selected Nathan's example as a case study to illustrate a slightly different perspective in a situation where all concerned were committed to giving Nathan the best care possible. Here, shared care and professional boundaries did not present a problem and collaboration between the PTC and the DGH worked well, yet we still see how problematic it can be to incorporate such specialised and extended palliative care into a general paediatric setting. Nathan had cancer, and the lack of expertise in the administration of chemotherapy was an issue. However, from what both John and Wendy told me, there are many challenges to providing end of life care in such a setting where most children are short-stay patients who recover, and most deaths tend to result from acute trauma. As Wendy said the majority of patients 'come in ill, they get better, they go home', thus many of the issues in question would have applied whatever Nathan's medical condition had been if it was terminal. Similarly, the shortage of staff and limited time to engage, as reported by John, would have remained the same.

We recall the model at the start of this chapter, formulated by Ashby et al. (1991), which suggested a series of measures necessary for the improvement of managing end of life care for children in hospital. Yet, 20 years later, the findings from the TCT end of life care service evaluation (Grinyer and Barbarachild 2011) generated almost the same list of concerns and limitations. The resource needs identified by participants in the evaluation as needing attention are summarised as follows:

- a specialist in palliative and end of life care accessible at all times
- training in pain management and control
- advanced age-appropriate communication skills
- pre-bereavement and bereavement skills training
- improved communications between PTC and community-based services.

Emotional support for staff was also identified as a need – as Contro et al. (2004) say, caring for dying children is stressful and caring for dying teenagers no less so. This evaluation also identified the need for an age-specific end of life care pathway. Currently, TCT units draw on one of a variety of *Supportive Care Pathway* documents, which are used at the end of a patient's life on most units, but are not TYA-specific. Most participants reported that some version of an adult end of life care pathway was adapted, including:

- the Liverpool Care Pathway (LCP) (2010)
- the 'University Hospital Board's' (UHB) policy

- a pathway based on the ACT Guidelines (normally for neuro-disability)
- a children's care pathway adapted for use with the TYAs. (Grinyer and Barbarachild 2011: 5)

The data presented here suggest that outside the specialist care setting of, for example, a paediatric cancer ward, palliative and end of life care are not managed well in the general hospital in either the paediatric or adult settings. The staff may be unfamiliar with end of life care, specialist care pathways may not be available, both adult and paediatric settings can be inappropriate – particularly for adolescents and young adults, communication with families and parents can be difficult, and collaboration between different specialisms can break down. That the hospital experience is less than satisfactory echoes the literature (e.g. Contro et al. 2004; Brook et al. 2006; Davis 2009) and the lack of expertise, limited emotional support, shortage of staffing and professional boundaries all add to the challenge experienced by staff and parents and their children.

Where end of life care does appear to work, there has been an element of fluidity between services, including hospice staff attending the child at the hospital, a TCT consultant accompanying the young patient to ICU, a local doctor's familiarity with a specialist centre and cooperation between a PTC and the DGH. The implications for policy and practice will be considered further in Chapter 6, but suffice it to say at this point that although there are examples of good practice, much hospital care leaves parents feeling that the end of their child's life could and should have been managed better.

Lessons for best practice

The experiences of the families, young people and professionals presented in this chapter suggest that there is much to be done to improve the incorporation of palliative and end of life care into hospital provision for children and young people. Many hospital environments focus on the treatment rather than the palliative care of children and young people, and as such may not have either the specialised clinical skills or training in emotional support to provide the best service. Based on the data collected in this chapter, there follows a list of suggestions to improve provision:

- Improved communication both between services and with parents and young people.
- Access to/development of specialist care pathways tailored to the needs and age group of the child or young person in question.
- Assurances that every care is taken to avoid infection for both cohorts.
- Shared care arrangements between the PTC and the DGH need to be improved, resources therefore need to be put into fostering relationships that transcend professionals' boundaries in preparation for shared care.

- A multi-disciplinary team based in the PTC can be instrumental in ensuring continuity of care.
- Paediatric wards need to be able to provide more age-appropriate settings and be willing to relinquish their care of the young person when appropriate.
- Transition between paediatric and adult care settings needs to be managed better - the potential gap in services for 16–18-year-olds in some areas must be addressed.
- Young adults who find themselves on wards with much older patients may need special consideration and sensitivity about where they are placed.
- Families need a key worker to liaise between the professionals and the family and patient, to avoid the impression that care is impersonal and their child's needs are not understood.
- Staff need appropriate training and support to manage the palliative and end of life care of children and young adults, particularly in the DGH where expertise in this area may be limited.

Chapter 5
Preparation for the End of Life, Bereavement and Emotional Support

This chapter moves away from care settings to consider the challenges facing both parents and professionals when treatment options fail and care becomes palliative, and examines how this is, or is not, discussed between the family, the young person and professionals, and how models of good practice can be applied in reality. It also considers how bereavement may be shaped by such interactions prior to the death and what support structures are available to bereaved families in their loss. A privileged glimpse of how parents interact in a bereavement support group is provided in order that both families and professionals, who may have little experience of such a group, can see how parents and other family members use such a forum as part of the grieving process.

As we saw in Chapter 1, preparation for bereavement is an essential part of the grieving process and most parents say they would have benefited from more preparatory information prior to their child's death (Contro and Scofield 2006). However, this involves not only the parents' own preparation for their impending loss but also the preparation of the young person for their death – what to tell them, how much and when. To some extent this will depend on the cognitive abilities of the young person, their age, maturity and willingness to engage in such interactions. However, when the parents try to protect their son or daughter and the son or daughter tries to do the same for their parents, the issue may never be addressed overtly but remain implicit. In my earlier research on how families of teenagers and young adults (TYAs) with cancer managed the sharing of medical information and prognoses with their sons and daughters (Grinyer 2002a), it became clear that a variety of strategies were used, from open and frank discussions between all parties in full knowledge of the situation, to parents shielding their son or daughter from the truth despite them being over the age of majority and consent. The rationale for concealment was that if the bleakness of the outlook was known, aggressive treatment might be refused, thus making survival even less likely. The range of approaches adopted is defined by the different awareness contexts listed as follows by ACT (2011c: 14)

- **closed awareness**: the child is not aware of the diagnosis, and those who know conceal it
- **suspected awareness**: the child is suspicious something is wrong, but is not certain
- **mutual pretence**: the child, family and health workers all know, but no one talks about it
- **open awareness**: everyone knows and is open about it.

There may be tacit acceptance that death is first a possibility, and ultimately an inevitability, with a continuum along which parents have to make decisions about what to divulge and when. However, this will also be shaped by the possibility of understanding intellectually, although having not accepted emotionally, that a child will die. Silverman (2000: 114) says that this 'knowing and not knowing' is a common phenomenon when faced with such a devastating prospect. During the course of their illness the young person may mature from being a child, when parents make the decisions and manage information, to being an adult who, in legal terms at least (see previous chapter for UK legal definition from ACT (2011c)), should be both the recipient of information and the decision maker. This sensitive situation may be even more problematic for children with cognitive disabilities, and judgements have to be made about how much they are able to understand and about how fully they can be included in decisions about their care and their future. Thus, we have a continually changing situation in terms of the illness trajectory, the child's developmental trajectory and parents' ability to accept the likelihood that their child will die; all these dynamics run concurrently and can be confusing for both the family and professionals.

A case study from the USA of Carrie, a 17-year-old girl with terminal cancer, is used by Turkoski (2003) to demonstrate the ethical and legal dilemmas facing health professionals when a parent forbids disclosure. In this instance, Carrie's mother issued orders to all her friends, family and health care providers that under no circumstances was her daughter to be told she had only a few weeks to live. Her mother refused to leave Carrie alone with anyone in case they 'let it slip' and made many comments such as 'when you get better'. Turkoski reports the negative impact this had on Carrie: she repeatedly asked why no one would talk to her about whether she would die and became taciturn and withdrawn as a result. The nurses caring for Carrie experienced what Turkoski calls 'professional pain' at violating their professional code and avoided her questions in order to steer clear of lying. From a legal standpoint, this case occurred in a US state where 'children under 18 have no legal rights to specific knowledge or participation in medical decision-making unless they are emancipated, in the armed services or married' (Turkoski 2003: 82). But Turkoski argues that the denial of reality makes children vulnerable and denies them the right to closure: the additional burden is placed on them of playing the game of 'not knowing'.

Discussing a child's imminent death with him or her is an extremely painful prospect (Kushnik 2010). The desire to spare the child anxiety and to avoid impairing the quality of life remaining may, according to Kushnik, give 'justifiable pause'. Death, she argues, is a term that can be synonymous with the 'evils' from which we want to protect our children and there may be a fear that to tell a child that he or she might die could result in them giving up and stopping their 'fight for life'. In conjunction with uncertain prognoses and lack of knowledge about how much a child can understand, this can lead to children remaining ignorant of the likelihood of their death. Kushnik also argues that the feeling that a child's death is such a tragic waste of life can act as a deterrent from making the death as 'good' as it can be. Indeed, the idea that it might be in any way positive could be considered distasteful.

Yet Kushnik reports surveys that suggest that the child may detect their parents' non-disclosure of their impending death, and as a result may lose trust in their parents and health care providers. If, as Kushnik says, a 'good death' is thought to include choice, preparation for death and leaving a legacy, these can only be achieved if the dying person has awareness of their imminent death. Knowing death is near is not, as Kushnik points out, the same as depriving the child of hope, as the loss of hope for an extended life does not mean there cannot be hope for a meaningful life and a good death. The use of advance care planning documents for adolescents and young adults is the focus of a study by Wiener et al. (2008), who observe that although discussions about the end of life with any population are difficult, with adolescents and young adults it is even more challenging and requires developmentally appropriate language. Nevertheless, these authors claim that young people in this age group express a strong desire to share in medical decision making and argue that it is their health care professionals and parents who find it difficult to initiate the conversation, as they fear it will counteract the 'culture of hope' central to paediatric and adolescent medical settings.

Alderson (1992) argues that competence is better understood when seen in the social context of a child's life, and that relying on their parents' estimation of their child's competence works only if the child and the parents agree, but becomes a crucial issue if they disagree. Alderson cites research showing that children as young as 5 can have a profound understanding of death. However, McCallum, Byrne and Bruera (2000), who undertook a study of children dying in a hospital setting, report that of their sample of 77, in only one case was there open communication with the dying patient (a teenager) despite the fact that their sample included seven 'cognitively intact' children over the age of 6. These authors suggest that children as young as 3 can have a rudimentary comprehension that they are dying even if they have not been told this. In a booklet designed by the Children's Cancer and Leukaemia Group (CCLG, 2007) to help parents whose child has a non-curable illness, there is an acknowledgment that a child's understanding of death depends on their 'spiritual beliefs, age and experience', but many children know 'deep down' when they are going to die: the problem is finding a way to talk about it.

It may be assumed that the comprehension of children with intellectual disabilities, who also have a life-limiting illness, is too limited for there to be any merit in addressing end of life care issues with them. Indeed, a search of the literature yielded nothing when looking for material specifically designed to address this issue with children who have cognitive impairment. To ensure I had missed nothing, I consulted Professor Chris Hatton an expert in the area, who confirmed that he knew of no publications or research that focused on this issue (pers. comm.). Several professionals I consulted at children's hospices also did not know of any such publications. However, although not aimed specifically at children or young people, two publications by CHANGE[1] (2010a, 2010b), one for people with learning disabilities and one for their carers, both address issues around end of life care and advance care planning. The version designed for people with learning disabilities includes an illustrated guide to what advance care planning entails and offers a very clear explanation of the options that may be available at the end of life; this might be suitable for some children and young people with cognitive problems or intellectual disabilities. Nevertheless, it seems that further research in this area would be helpful in generating material that could be of assistance to both parents and professionals in this difficult task.

The bereavement needs of families

So, it seems that the whole context of a child's death is fraught with challenges about the 'right' way to manage it. For the surviving parents, the bereavement process may be shaped by how their child's death was managed, in terms of the appropriateness of medical interventions and the place of death – which as we have seen can be crucial – and how the communication of important end of life issues was managed. To regret not having been able to say 'goodbye', or not having shared the truth with a lost son or daughter, can make the grieving process even more difficult. Rosenblatt (2000: 49) argues that the last minutes spent with a dying child are 'often filled with awe and with emotional pain'. These last moments have the potential for immense and lasting significance and can, Rosenblatt argues, be done 'beautifully or horribly, gracefully or clumsily, with love and controlled caring or with chaos'. Rosenblatt reports some parents as saying these last minutes contained a clear message that the end was near and offered the opportunity for a final 'goodbye'.

Kushnik (2010) cites a Swedish study that suggests that those parents who discussed their child's imminent death with them had a much less complicated bereavement process, whereas 27% of those who had not discussed it later regretted this. Parents who 'sensed' their child was aware of their impending death but still did not address it with them directly, expressed a higher level of post-death regret at nearly 50%. None of the parents who had discussed their impending death with their child reported regretting this.

[1] CHANGE is an organisation that works to advance human rights and equality for people with learning disabilities.

Whatever choices have been made by parents during their child's illness and end of life care – whether or not they have been able to share full information with their child – the bereavement that follows their loss is a crucial stage during which, with appropriate support at the right time, families can learn to rebuild their lives. However, it seems that many professionals involved in the support and care of the child through illness and death either do not see their role as extending beyond the death or are unsure of how and when to offer appropriate post-death interventions. Before I began my research with bereaved parents, I spoke to health professionals about what it would be helpful for them to know about the bereavement process. I was asked by them to discover if parents would welcome the attendance of their child's health carers at the funeral; whether parents would welcome ongoing contact with their child's health care professionals; when it would be appropriate to engage the parents in a bereavement programme; what such bereavement support might look like; would parents welcome joining a group with other bereaved parents? Although these questions were intended to 'inform' the research process, they were also in themselves 'findings' and indicated a lack of security relating to the professionals' own understanding of their role and their uncertainty about how to engage with a patient's family after death. To some extent this was associated with the setting of care, the hospital staff being less sure about the process than hospice staff. However, the relative certainty of the hospice staff did not necessarily translate into interventions or result in the type of support experienced by bereaved families as helpful, thus in some cases suggesting a model of grief that did not meet individuals' needs.

There is much literature on the grieving process and on how to support family members post bereavement (e.g. Rosenblatt 2000; Silverman 2000; Field and Behrman 2003; Baker McCall 2004; Berzoff and Silverman 2004). Baker McCall (2004) says grieving can be described as a journey and she says that the grief process, like a journey, has a beginning, a middle and an end with several stages: shock and numbness, denial, feelings, depression, reorganisation and recovery (Baker McCall 2004: 47). As Baker McCall says, there are numerous variations of this model but this one, based on 'solid theory and research', is clinically useful as it is associated with positive outcomes. However, she says, grief can be complicated, needing allowances to be made for the uniqueness of each person; it can also be what Baker McCall defines as 'dysfunctional' and considered pathological. Baker McCall points out that a consensus regarding the terminology has yet to be reached, thus the situation is complex for professionals engaged in the support and treatment of those who are grieving. Referrals can be made for 'complicated' grief even when the grief is 'normal', and grieving may be considered 'dysfunctional' even if an individual is functioning well. But in this book we are considering the grief over the loss of a child. Although the death of anyone with whom there has been a meaningful relationship will result in grief and feelings of loss, the death of a child at any age challenges our assumptions about the 'natural order' of life and death, as in contemporary Western society we do not expect our children to predecease us (Sourkes 1977; Milo 1997). It is arguable that the impact of the death of a child will have a different quality: indeed,

I began this book with a sentence that contained the words 'there is something profoundly "wrong" about a child predeceasing its parents'.

According to Field and Behrman (2003: 11), after the death of a child most of the bereavement support comes from 'friends, neighbors, spiritual advisers, hospice personnel, grief counselors and others in the community'. However, it is acknowledged that the clinical staff who cared for the child can 'be with' the family in a meaningful way following the death, and that an abrupt end to the parents' relationship with those who cared for their son or daughter can feel like abandonment. As a result, it is suggested that hospitals where children die should work with hospices and community organisations, to help identify and coordinate culturally sensitive bereavement services, define the bereavement support roles for both hospital-based and non-hospital personnel and respond to the bereavement needs of professionals as well as families.

Macdonald et al. (2005) suggest that after the death of a child, acts of kindness by staff who cared for the child and their family are highly significant. Receiving cards and telephone calls and attendance at the funeral by staff were all valued and remembered by bereaved parents. Disappointment was expressed when staff failed to follow-up in these ways. However, Macdonald et al. also suggest that parents can find it difficult to return to the hospital where their child was cared for, as this is too painful. Nevertheless, all the parents in their study had attended a memorial service at the hospital, some finding closure in their return. Some comments suggested that it showed they were not alone in their loss, demonstrated that the staff cared and that the reading of names and lighting of candles were all significant symbolic acts. In contrast, some parents found it emotionally draining, others had felt they had no choice but to attend, and some felt disappointed if they did not see staff they recognised at the service. Thus, it seems that the experience can be 'bittersweet' and unpredictable.

Rosenblatt (2000) says that at the core of the support parents found the most valuable was 'non-judgemental' listening and constancy. The support from people who had experienced similar losses was also valued as it validated bereaved parents' continuing pain and bond to their lost child. Thus, a support group of other parents who have experienced the loss of a child may not only validate what might be perceived by others as dysfunctional grief, but also can foster relationships between members that transcend the group and the discussion of the loss. There can be a tacit acceptance of similar experiences without the continuing need to discuss them explicitly.

We now move on to examine how these issues are experienced and managed, through the personal accounts of both bereaved parents and staff who have cared for dying children.

Findings

The empirical data used in this chapter are derived from both studies - thus, there is material about children with complex life-limiting conditions and TYAs with cancer. However, although the hospice evaluation study included end of life care issues where this was relevant, it was primarily about long-term palliative care with families whose children's life expectancy was unpredictable. Thus, the first part of the *Findings* section of this chapter on communicating with a son or daughter about their approaching death is drawn from the TYA study, whereas the second part on the parents' preparation for bereavement and the emotional needs of the families post bereavement draws on both studies.

When curative becomes palliative: the difficulties of disclosure

For some of the young people with severe cognitive impairments, the situation may appear to be comparatively straightforward in that it is assumed they do not have the ability to comprehend their own death. Although for some this may be the case, the publications for people with learning disabilities mentioned above (CHANGE 2010a, 2010b) may provide a vehicle to address the issue with those children and young people with whom it is appropriate. Nevertheless, in the hospice service evaluation there was no evidence that end of life care had been addressed with the children and young people in question. This seems to have been partly because it was difficult to know when the palliative treatment they had been in receipt of all their lives moved into the end of life phase, and partly because many had severe cognitive difficulties that may have made such a discussion seem inappropriate. In contrast, for the TYAs with cancer it is usually the case that they are capable of understanding fully the implications of their illness, and the transition from treatment to end of life is care is more identifiable. Yet, in all instances, individual family dynamics shape the process of disclosure. For example, parents' assumptions about their son's or daughter's ability and willingness to be open about their prospects of survival, their age and cognitive ability, maturity, the certainty or otherwise of the prognosis, all influence the decisions parents make about telling their children that their care has become palliative and that treatment is no longer curative. This can be problematic for professionals who may make judgements according to the chronological age of the patient and assume that he or she 'should' have been told or will already be aware of the situation.

An instance of how miscommunication can damage relationships between parents and professionals is demonstrated in the following example. Clare's son, Joe, died when he was 20, yet she had been told at regular intervals from when he was diagnosed at 13 with anaplastic astrocytoma (a type of brain tumour), that he would die. In the intervening 7 years, Joe had undergone a series of crises, any one of which could have heralded his death. As Clare said, she could have told Joe at any time during that period that he would die; this is her rationale for not doing so:

> It wasn't as if ... We weren't lying to him. You know, if he'd have asked those questions, whatever he asked we were honest with him all the way through. I wouldn't tell him that he's going to get better ... We might say ...

"Well we just don't know", and that was the truth of it to be honest, because we didn't know, because we were told so many times that he was really ill and he got over it, and he was well ... In the end you think, well you don't know who to believe ...
(Clare)

However, Clare's careful protection of Joe against being told he might die was threatened when he was admitted to an adult hospital ward where the consultant disagreed with her approach. The way she tells the story of her first encounter with this consultant suggests an attitude and approach that Clare found inappropriate:

We went up to the adults' ward and Joe was up there, and he was very, very poorly but he weren't deaf ... you know, he was just in bed. And he was all there [in] his mind ... he'd been there a couple of days and then this [consultant], she came up to the ward and she said, "Have you told him he's dying?" And he was laying in the bed. He was asleep ... and I went, "Excuse me ..." ... I just remember [saying] "shh, shh" you know. She whispers, "Have you told him that he's dying?" ... I've never met the woman ... never met her before. I said, "No", I said, "and nor will we". You know, I said, "We won't ... there's no reason for us to ..." "He should be told" she said, "because he knows you know". I said, "How do you know he knows?" she said, "Because I know". She said, "I know that he knows". She said, "I know that they know". And I said, "Well, if he knew then he wouldn't be talking about when he comes out of hospital – he wants to do this and when he comes out he wants to do that". I said, "If he knew he wouldn't be speaking that way". I said, "And until he asks a question like that ... I can't see any reason that we need to tell him". She disagreed and I don't think she particularly liked me after that, because she disagreed with the way that we ... that we felt that he didn't need ... you know why did you need ...why did he need to know?
(Clare)

Joe was 20, would have been able to understand what he was told, and the consultant might have been correct in her assumption that he 'knew'; yet it may be that Joe did not want to 'know' and deliberately chose to ignore the implications of his worsening health. Whatever the 'rights and wrongs' of this situation, the distress caused by this bedside encounter could have been avoided with better communication and understanding between the parents and the consultant.

In a slightly different scenario, we have evidence of a young person's reluctance to confront his impending death in the case of Ian, a young American, who died at 23 from oesophageal cancer. He resisted all attempts by both his parents and health care professionals to address his approaching death. The following is an extract from my interview with Ian's mother and father, Laura and Arthur:

Laura:

We ... never really talked with Ian about anything other than his treatments and what lay in store for him as far as what he needed to do to get well ... he didn't want to talk about those things. Nobody ever that I know of brought it up, you know, that this wasn't gonna be as positive an outcome as we had hoped ... so, no, we never, we never really ... we touched on it a little ... we never really, never really addressed what did he want, how did he want to do it - all he wanted to talk about was what his options were for treatments and, and, you know, working towards hopefully a cure.

AG:

Do you think he accepted that he might not survive?

Laura:

I tussle with that all the time, because I wasn't able to really get a clear idea. He was very smart, very, very intelligent, and I know he knew odds very well ... and I know that his goal was - he told me from the beginning when he was first diagnosed, that weekend, that "I'm gonna beat this, I'm gonna beat this." ... And then I think he focused all his energy on that and never really talked to anybody. He spent a great deal of time with my husband, going back and forth to treatment. I would be at work and meet them there ... but they spent a lot of time alone together in the car, on the ride, and ... while he was having his chemo or ... his fluids. And you didn't speak about it all ...

Arthur:

No - but when the doctors told him he was dying he said he didn't want to deal with it, he refused to deal with it. I think he refused to accept it.

Laura:

Right up to the end ... about ... a week before he died, he was admitted to the hospital with ... a bad cough and what looked like pneumonia, and ... his nurse said, "You know you can stay here until you pass" and he was kind of in and out in that kind of ... I don't know if it was a drug-induced or ... the cancer was ... just rapidly diminishing him, but he said: "What do you mean 'pass'?" and she said, "When you die?" He said, "I'm dying?" And he said ... what was his quote?

Arthur:

"I can't cope, deal with this."

Laura:

"I can't deal with this" ... yeah, and he just ... he kind of was in and out, in and out, in and out after that ... so we never really ... touched on anything, you know, what ... what did he want, what did he hope for? ... none of that.

> **AG:**
> Do you, do you think that that made his end of life care more difficult in some ways, that you weren't addressing it overtly?
>
> **Laura:**
> Absolutely ... absolutely, it made it impossible because you were on eggshells all the time, not knowing if you were doing the right thing or the wrong thing. He was very polite. One of the things that you talked to anybody that dealt with him at the hospital, any of nursing staff: "What a polite, pleasant, well-mannered young man ..." He never had any kind of hostile attitude towards anybody. He was always sweet as pie ... you just didn't want to push him one way or the other and take his control away. He was in charge of making his decisions: we were there ... as much as we could be, which was a lot of the time, most of the time ... whenever there was a discussion between the doctors and him, we were there. On a few occasions they, they would ask us to leave the room ... 21 is the legal age in America and he was ... 22 when he was diagnosed so ... you know, we respected that, but I think – he never actually said it – but he would allude to ... that he didn't want to hear all the ... fine stuff.

Ian was offered the opportunity to remain in hospital where his parents had faith that his end of life care would be well managed, that he would be kept pain-free and he would not choke to death as was their great fear. However, Ian insisted on going home – whether this was based on a desire to die at home is not clear, as the prospect of his death was never addressed overtly. Despite their misgivings, Ian's parents conceded to his wish to be discharged to hospice support at home (see Chapter 2). Ian's case raises a number of issues about young adults' right to make a choice – even though that choice may be against medical advice and their parents' better judgement. This in turn raises the question of whether parents should try to insist on what they perceive to be the 'safer' option in light of their greater experience, or whether they should allow their young adult child the autonomy to make their own decisions and possibly their own mistakes.

Although it may be understandable that the clinician caring for Joe at 20 would assume he did know or 'ought to' know his prognosis, Karen told me how the seriousness of her son Mason's condition was conveyed to him at only 13:

> And Mason's consultant ... I mean, bearing in mind ... he was only just 13 ... she just spun round in her chair and she just said, "Mason your tumour's bad, and boy have you got a fight on your hands this time".
> (Karen)

Karen said she was unsure of the extent to which Mason understood the implications of this comment, but she was so shocked by it that it shaped how his parents managed all subsequent consultations:

After that initial consultation we never, ever took Mason with us to any consultations until we went first ... because we just felt that the way they dealt with it there and then ... all right, he was a teenager, but we had no idea they were going to say that to us. So we couldn't even take it onboard. To have him there sitting with us, and not knowing what they were going to say each time we saw them ... I mean, when they called us in to tell us about his treatment, we didn't take him with us and they said the treatment was going to be absolutely horrendous. We had to sign to say that he could have a heart attack, he could go deaf, blah, blah, blah, each time before he had his treatment. We didn't want him knowing all that.
(Karen)

The way the end of Mason's life was managed is related by Karen as follows:

They just called George and I in on the 26th of March and just said, "There's nothing more we can do for him. It's getting bigger; it's in his lungs and it's travelling to his brain". We didn't tell Mason what the news was, but we then had to have this whole team coming in who Mason wasn't aware of, or knew, and it just made it so hard, because as far as they were aware, they were the end of life team – so this child that they were dealing with should know that he was at the end of his life, because it would make their job a lot easier ... And I know they deal with teenagers, and some parents opt for that choice. But the day they told us that there was no more they could do for Mason, he was actually at school. So we wasn't going to bring him home from school [and say] "Oh, guess what ..." ... He died on the 30th of April, so it was only 4 weeks after that date. And for 2 weeks of that he was good; he was very, very good. And we were the bravest we've ever had to be in those 2 weeks. As Mason became more in pain we knew it was coming closer, so therefore he was becoming sedated more ... There was a point, the weekend Mason died, when he just said to his dad, "I can't take this life anymore. I can't do this anymore". They say that Mason knew something was happening then. Whether he didn't say anything to us because he didn't want to frighten us, or he didn't want to hear it, we don't know ... I don't think Mason knew he was going to die, because I think he would have been terrified. I think he would have been absolutely terrified. And we didn't know how long we had left with Mason, and I couldn't bear the thought of every time that boy shut his eyes, you didn't know if he was going to wake up again. And I couldn't bring myself to say it. And as far as I was concerned, while he was breathing he was alive and there was a chance. You know, you do hear of stories where people are told they've got a week to live, you know ... And I just ... I couldn't ... I just wanted him to do as much as he could for as long as he could, without him thinking, "Well I'm going to die" ...
(Karen)

Karen's account makes it very clear how difficult a parent finds it to tell a child that they are dying, motivated by their hope that the prognosis may be wrong and the desire to spare their child what they believe will be terror at the prospect of death. In Chapter 4 we learned that Amy, at 13, the same age as Mason, had Asperger's syndrome and as a result did not understand the concept of death. Her parents therefore took the decision not to tell her she was unlikely to wake up from the general anaesthetic she was to be given – what she thought of as her 'magic sleep'. As her mother Pam told the doctors, "I don't want Amy to know she's not going to wake up" ... and they [the doctors] said, "No, I think that's understandable" ... It was so hard. It was so hard to make that decision ...' (Pam). So here we have an example of the professionals involved in Amy's case being supportive of her parents' approach. The rationale for this is apparent; Pam was deemed justified in concealing the truth because of Amy's cognitive limitations. However, the literature (McCallum, Byrne and Bruera 2000, CHANGE 2010a, 2010b) suggests that both very young children and those with learning difficulties may have the ability to grasp the concept of death and have the right to make choices. Yet it is also possible to imagine how problematic such negotiations and communication would be under the distressing circumstances surrounding end of life care decision making – particularly for a child who has always been protected by their parents. However, for those children and young people deemed to have the cognitive ability to comprehend their own death, the majority of the health professionals were adamant that it was essential that they be fully informed of the prognosis, as Saul the Director of Day and Out Patient Services at an adult hospice, sums up:

> So long as you're communicating and you're communicating as honestly as you can, I think you minimise the long-term problem. You might not minimise the short term, but that kind of denial or lying to children causes far more problems in the long term. When you have youngsters, teenagers or young adults, they have enough cognitive ability to very quickly sound you out, they know when you're bullshitting them. They're very quick to feel someone is trustworthy or untrustworthy and, for better or worse, I always approach care of those individuals and their families in a sometimes quite brutally honest manner, but as sensitively as I possibly can.
> (Saul)

Nevertheless, however 'brutally honest' or sensitive the approach, the acceptance of a terminal diagnosis may not be straightforward. In Bianca's account of her husband Ryan's prognosis it is evident that although they had been told unequivocally that Ryan – nearly 22 – would die, neither was able to take this in at a meaningful level. Although they heard and 'understood' at a cognitive level, they were unable to accept it emotionally. As Bianca said:

> I remember when our Nurse Consultant sat us all down and said, you know, "You've got the ... three months, you need to take it in". I remember him taking me outside going, "That's a crock of shit, it's not gonna happen. Don't worry, I know how strong I am", and he never, never sort of ... ever said out loud, he never admitted he was gonna die – so much so he never made a will, he never made any provisions for dying because I just think it was too hard for him ... I think he needed to live with this kind of, "I'm gonna be okay", because I think the thought of death ... I think for all of us was horrendous ... I know that when I married him I hoped against hope he'd get better. I know right up until the morning that he died, that in my head I genuinely believed something would happen that would save him ... When he did die it was a complete shock ... it took me ... a week to actually get my head around what had happened.
> (Bianca)

In Bianca's account we can see that although the professionals were explicit, and indeed she recalls them being explicit, the reality of Ryan's impending death was unimaginable and therefore remained unreal. Thus, the 'knowing but not knowing' (Silverman 2000) can clearly apply not only to parents but also to the young people. Ryan, an educated young man of almost 22, could have been considered well able to understand and 'accept' the prognosis – yet at this age why should the prospect of death seem either acceptable or reasonable? Thus, even in an 'open awareness' context nothing can be assumed about the ability to accept death as inevitable. This was reiterated by the palliative nurse specialist Anne, who said:

> What we have to remember is somebody of that age group, no matter how much you spell it out to them, they cannot believe that their life's coming to an end. Even though they may verbalise that they under-stand – which they do – there's that actual thing: "I'm too young to die".
> (Anne)

There is a middle ground between concealment and an open awareness context in which the expectation of death remains implicit and unspoken; it falls somewhere between 'suspected awareness' and 'mutual pretence' (ACT 2011c: 14). An example is shown in the following account from Joan of the last 10 days of her son Stuart's life:

> One night he just said to me, "Mum, I've had enough. I've had enough of this". He ... was going into the bathroom and he was on his hands and knees because he was too wobbly on his legs. And he just said to me, "I've had enough now". And you know I thought he was going to die that night. I must admit, I didn't sleep at all that night. I just sat beside him because he was so poorly, and I thought he's never going to make it out of here. But, you know typical of Stuart fashion, he managed to rally and

... [they] offered him more chemotherapy. By that time he couldn't even sit in a wheelchair, it was too uncomfortable. And he just said, "No" ... It [was] his way of saying ... "If it happens it happens, I don't want any more of that stuff". It never came to the point where we had to have "the conversation". You see, Stuart had been to funerals, so he knew. I mean, we'd been to a boy's funeral in March of the year that he died, you know, and he didn't look very well then. But you know, he just said to me at the funeral – because the mum ... was really, really distraught ... because she was hysterical, you know, just quite shocking – and he said to me, "Mum, don't ever do that to me, will you?" and I said, "No mate, I wouldn't do that to you".
(Joan)

Despite all the unspoken communication between Stuart and his mother that his death was likely, she said the following about what happened when his condition worsened suddenly and rapidly:

I just ... dialled 999, "He's not breathing!". And then he started to breathe again, and the ambulance came, and they sort of sorted him out a bit. And they were going to take him off to hospital ... I mean, he came down the chair ... down the stairs on a chair. He wasn't on a bed or anything. And he just said to me, "Don't worry mum, I'll be alright" and that's the last thing he ever said.
(Joan)

Rosie told me a similar story about her son Hugh, with whom she had never had an explicit conversation about his possible death, although it seems she suspected that he was aware his condition was terminal. However, Hugh had visited a therapist in whom Rosie believed he might have confided concerns about his death, Rosie said:

He never actually spoke about it to me. You would have to speak about it to his psychotherapist, upon whom he unloaded. But he didn't talk to anybody else until days before the end really ... He was in a coma for the last 3 or 4 days, and in the last week one or the other of us had been sleeping up in his room. And he certainly ... was very high on morphine at this stage, and he said to my daughter, "I can't go to sleep because he's going to get me". And he said in the morning, "He didn't get me". So, he was aware in the last week that he was dying. I mean he was aware before that but ...
(Rosie)

Ellen was 23 when she died; her mother Ann said the following about her unwillingness to talk about her death and her belief that if she stayed in hospital there might still be hope:

> I think she realised nothing else could be done. So I think she knew that was what was going to happen. She still didn't want to talk about it … because when she was in hospital in London she was always desperate to get home … Even when she really wasn't well enough to be home she'd bargain with her consultant, you know, "Can I go now?" … "Well if I'm good today, can I go tomorrow?" … She'd just want to be home basically. And for the first time she didn't actually want to go home. But she didn't want to stay there – I know she didn't want to stay there – but maybe she just thought they could somehow find something that would sort everything out, you know.
> (Ann)

Although Hugh, Stuart and Ellen were all significantly older when they died, Beckie, the mother of Billie who died at 14, described a similarly ambiguous situation. Beckie felt Billie knew she was dying, and yet at another level she perhaps had not quite grasped what that meant:

> We think they understand … or we think they don't understand. We don't really know how much they understand because they're children … you know, I'm talking about Billie, she was 14 … but she knew she was going to die, and we kind of thought she knew it was soon. But she didn't really … I think we did all the right things in a lot of people's minds, but that's because it was right for us, not because I'd read a book and somebody had told me it was the right thing … I mean I do think that people should not be rigid, because I have heard of parents being told that they really must tell their child that they're going to die … No, don't tell somebody what they should do with their child – just don't.
> (Beckie)

This final sentence 'don't tell somebody what they should do with their child – just don't', perhaps sums up on behalf of all the families just how sensitive health professionals need to be to the individual dynamics between parents and their dying children. Few assumptions can be made about the correlation between the chronological age of the child and their capacity and competence, and their legal right to be informed and make choices. Sarah, a clinician with a great deal of experience with young people who have cancer and also other life-limiting conditions, commented on the difficulty many young people have in addressing the reality of their terminal condition:

> The consultant would certainly have the frank discussions with the family that the treatment isn't working and that that young person is now terminal. So the young person would be included in those discussions. In my experience, I've often found that the young people actually don't want to accept that, and that even when you've told them that their condition is terminal … they'll go on the internet, they'll research new drugs, they'll want to look at new treatments, and then they will go back to the

consultants and ask whether it's possible to have further treatment. That's when I think that it has to be led by the young person. You have to give them the opportunities to talk about death and dying, if they want to, and that's obviously open-ended conversations with them, to ask them how they're feeling about the information that they've been given, have they got any questions, is there anything that you can help them with or any particular things that they would like you to do for them? But I have often found that the young people, they don't always want to engage with you and talk about death and dying, but that's at a point when they will want to go out more with their friends if they're capable of doing that, and they perhaps might want to book that holiday. They could be really poorly but will still want to do that holiday … I remember a young lady that I worked with, she made the decision that she wanted to bring forward her 18th birthday party and have a party with her friends before she died. She wanted to plan her funeral, her music and she did a lot of the writing that she wanted read out at her funeral. But I think that's unusual … In my experience, a large percentage of the young adults don't want to talk about death and dying, and they want to live as full a life as possible if they can until the end.
(Sarah)

In some cases the need to plan their funeral is important to the young person, but can also be significant to their loved ones after the death. Sue B, the Clinical Nurse manager at an adult hospice where age-appropriate provision for teenagers and young adults from 14 upwards was being developed, said:

And if you've done your very best for that person while they're alive and then suddenly you don't know whether they want to be buried or cremated, you don't know what songs they wanted … you're left with that "Well, I didn't do my best" … so it's just so vital that we do talk about these things and that we do get people to express their wishes, to enable the person that's living to continue to live afterwards.

One of the questions asked on the referral form, "Is the patient and the family aware of the reasons for referral?" … because … when you make contact and say, "I'm the nurse from the hospice, the doctor referred you to our services", some people are quite shocked. So although GPs (general practitioners) or oncologists may think it's the right thing to do, sometimes they haven't been quite as explicit as they could be with the patient themselves. So we've got to be very tentative in how we say, "Hello", you know, "I'm from the hospice, I don't know if you're aware but your doctor (or your nurse consultant, or whoever the referrer is) made a referral to our services. Are you okay with that?" … From the very outset, we're talking openly and we don't collude with people who say,

"Oh, please don't talk to my son or my daughter, I don't want you to talk about death and dying because it's too upsetting." ... If they should ask us a question we're only going to be truthful about that ... And sometimes they test you, [they ask], "Am I going to die then nurse?" ... They're judging your response to that by how you continue to work with that individual, because if you were to jolly that person along and say, "Oh well, we won't talk about that right now, that's a bit of a morbid subject. Let's carry on and ... what music would you like on?" ... You know you're going to bluff over things and you're going to jolly them along, and you've got to respect that they are individuals and they need the truth ... To be jollied along and cajoled into, "Oh well, let's take each day as it comes", or "Let's take it a day at a time", is not helpful to that person, because you've got to enable that person to have endings, to say goodbye, to have those meetings with people, make their peace, and make their memory boxes for others, talk about their experiences and things that have been good or bad for them in their lives, and maybe even plan for their own funeral, because they're still in control. You would expect someone 16-18-year-olds to have an understanding of life and death, whereas an 8-year-old may have only witnessed the death of a pet ... You would expect that - the normal developmental stages of any individual, by the time they're 16, they understand the concept of death and not being here anymore.

(Sue B)

Sue's response suggests that the accepted practice for patients of any age is extended to the younger age group as 'good practice'. What is perhaps surprising is the discrepancy between what is widely regarded as 'good practice' and how so many of the deaths recounted in this chapter have been managed. But the selected examples I have presented demonstrate how very difficult it is for parents to address their son's or daughter's impending death and that even in families where the truth has not been deliberately concealed, obfuscation and avoidance of the issue can occur.

The bereavement needs of parents and families

We begin this section by looking at the emotional and bereavement needs of the parents in the hospice service evaluation. All these parents had children who had experienced lifelong complex life-threatening illness and had thus in some senses been 'prepared' for the possibility of their early death since birth. However, such 'preparedness' does not constitute any formal pre-bereavement counselling rather just an underlying knowledge, or dread, that a child's life will be cut short. To live on a daily basis with the implicit prospect of such a loss places parents under continuous emotional stress. However, although parents did not expect hospice staff to provide emotional support for the 'everyday' impact, support was sought at particularly stressful times such as during a crisis, at the end of life and during bereavement.The ongoing emotional needs of the parents and wider families, which are not confined to events surrounding the end of life and post bereavement, are thus not always met. The psychosocial impact extends to all family members throughout the period they are supporting their children and grandchildren, as the case of a grandmother, Nora, illustrates. Nora regularly travelled some distance from her own home to stay with her daughter to help care for her baby grandson, Barnie; she clearly felt she was the lynchpin keeping the family together, but also felt isolated and without support herself:

> I feel a bit in the middle sometimes, I don't want to step on any toes, as you might say. But I am the one that holds it all together ... "Who hugs the nanas?" ... Because I haven't got a partner, if I hug [the family] then I am supporting them. But I need someone to hold me sometimes ... I used to come about once month for a few days. Since about 2 weeks before the end of the pregnancy, I have been home a few times. [I] always ... had to come rushing back ... I have had a couple of chest infections and had to go to bed for a week ... Or I go home. I dash around and put everything in order, and then I dash back again ... I hadn't been out for a coffee or out with a friend for at least 6 months. I have had one meal with one friend, and one cup of coffee with another friend since Barnie was born ... I also feel I am the kingpin that tries to hold it all together, but every now and then I have got to go home ... But I sleep in [Barnie's brother] Sam's room, so that does it even more so. When they go rushing to the hospital or to the hospice or whatever, it's me that tends to pick up the pieces with Sam who is sobbing his heart out that his brother is going to die.
> (Nora)

The social and emotional needs of this grandparent who feels herself to be the 'kingpin' without whom the family will not cope, appear to remain unmet. This may be because 'holding the fort' at home she is hidden from the view of those who might notice her need.

If signs that the child's life is ending become apparent, pre-bereavement support and counselling are clearly of importance. For example, Dan's stepmother Tania said the counselling service had been important to her in coping with the anticipatory grieving, prior to Dan's death when she was unable to stop crying. Tania met with the hospice staff about 6 months prior to Dan's death to discuss his end of life care needs, a process that was clearly integral to their preparing for his death emotionally as well as practically. As Tania said: 'The hospice prepared us better than the hospital, 6 months before the eventuality', thus suggesting that such support is more likely to be found in hospices than in a paediatric hospital care setting. However, despite their skill in preparing the family prior to the death, it seems that few assumptions can be made about when a family member will be 'ready' for post-bereavement support. Tania said her younger son, Nick, 'needed help urgently, but the [post-bereavement] play sessions didn't run for a few months. They like to let a few months go by first'. This indicates that support sessions for siblings can also be of great importance. However, the timing may have to be assessed on a case-by-case basis so that those in need of this type of intervention can access it sooner, if appropriate, as 'letting a few months go by' may leave some without much-needed support.

Whether the young person had died at the hospice, at home or in hospital, hospice services were experienced as supportive and inclusive. One of the options valued highly in the immediate aftermath of the death was being able to keep the deceased child's body at home, or alternatively using the cold room at the hospice for this purpose. When the family can be in shock and want to stay close to their lost child while saying 'goodbye', such an option can offer great comfort to parents whose child's body may otherwise be taken from them prematurely. If the 'special bedroom' at the hospice becomes familiar to families in advance of death, it can be a place of sanctuary and comfort where family and friends can spend time with the dead child before the funeral. However, the families' needs are ongoing, and they may require greater support as time progresses, as activity around the death recedes and as the permanence of their loss becomes real. Sheila described the need for flexibility in offering bereavement support:

> When a child's referred to us, they get put into a contact group partnership, and so those people would be phoning the family while the child was alive and negotiating when they want to come in or what's happening for them. And so, after the death, the same people would initially phone the family, unless they've come for their first stay and had never had any of that. And then, with the family, we would explain what services are available. And then, if they wanted them there and then, we would pass them on to the designated bereavement team. But they rotate on to that team, so they might even know them and they may have cared for the child. But then, throughout the year, we would maybe offer for them to come to our [memorial] service. Some families may say, "I don't want you to come and visit me, but when you have your [memorial] service I would like to be invited". And that might be a key point when they then want ... to take up bereavement services. Because everyone is different and I think you have to be a little bit flexible in how you offer it. And some people, it might be a year before they want it ... We always send an anniversary card ... What we've found is, for lots of the families, the first year there's huge hurdles and they feel really pleased they've got over those hurdles and expect to feel better in the second year. And in fact, in the second year, they feel worse because they thought it would be worse in the first year ... and it's now another year. And I think also the way in which death sometimes is treated, is people can forget about the child ... If all their peers, when they start university or are doing their A levels, it is really significant times of what your child isn't then doing. (Sheila)

Hospices appear to be well prepared to offer support to families whose child has died but the use of such services may be constrained by the proximity of the hospice to the family home. Liz from Douglas House in Oxford said:

> We are very involved in offering bereavement support to families ... and a new thing that we are increasingly using is peer support, so in other words workshops for bereaved families which may include other bereaved families ... taking part in that workshop or putting on that workshop. But also, just the support that they get from the other fairly recently bereaved parents ... that is absolutely incredibly helpful. But if you've got to travel all the way from Devon, Cornwall, Wales ... just for maybe a 3-hour workshop, the chances are quite high you're not going to do it – whereas if you live an hour's drive away, then you probably will make the effort to do it. So we found that we were not able to support people in the way that we wanted to, either the young people themselves as they went into a crisis, or the families after the death. So yes it is difficult if you're taking people too far away from home.
> (Liz)

Diane and Len had fostered 10 children with complex, multiple life-limiting conditions, all of whom were supported by their local hospice service. They had experienced a number of bereavements and spoke of the centrality of the hospice support services in the immediate aftermath and longer-term after the deaths, even though none of the children had actually died there. Diane said:

> The children that have died have not actually died at [the hospice] ... The first child that we lost, the [hospice] staff helped us keep him at home, helped us wash him and get him prepared, came every day and made sure that things were all right with us. They also supported us when we did move [him] into the funeral home, because that was prior to [the hospice] opening. Following that, the other two boys that died, they went straight to [the hospice] from the hospital, where they had died, and they helped us look after them there. We were included in everything that needed to be done there, until they left for the funeral ... Sometimes they will ring and say, would I mind speaking to a family who has either had a bereavement or who has just been diagnosed with something that might be similar to whatever, or something like that, and that is always OK.
> (Diane)

We can see from Diane's account that not only have she and her family been supported after the deaths of their foster children, they have also been asked to support others in a similar position, which as Rosenblatt (2000) says can be a great source of comfort for bereaved parents. Although Diane and Len seemingly received adequate bereavement care, an interview with Rosemarie from an adult hospice suggested that resources could be scarce and bereavement support limited as a consequence:

> We used to ... do a couple of bereavement visits and some phone calls but, resource-wise, we just don't have the facilities now. I think one bereavement phone call, the odd bereavement visit if it's sort of really, really needed ... We do have a bereavement group, and we have our bereavement service who are absolutely stretched to their limits.
> (Rosemarie)

Thus, input from other parents who have already been through the process, like Len and Diane, could act as an important resource helping not only the more recently bereaved but perhaps also as a therapeutic activity for those whose loss is less recent. However, if bereavement services are hard to provide through a hospice, counselling through another route – perhaps The Compassionate Friends – may be an alternative way to support family members under such circumstances. Nevertheless, it became clear that this is not an attractive option for everyone. For example, one mother said counselling had opened a 'can of worms' for her, so she had stopped it. Under such circumstances a more informal network, such as that offered through parents like Diane, may be preferable. For some, other kinds of support may be more acceptable than counselling. Brenda, for example, said she had not sought counselling from the hospice, even after a particularly stressful period when her son Nathan had been ill and in hospital; instead, she had been referred by the hospice for complementary therapies such as reflexology and massage for 6 weeks. This appeared to meet her needs better than perhaps the more 'obvious' strategy of formal counselling.

It is also important to recognise that the willingness to accept post-bereavement support from those who have been involved in the care of the lost son or daughter will be shaped by the trust and pre-existing relationship families have had with the service. For example – drawing on the TYA study – Laura, whose experience of the home-based hospice service (see Chapter 2) in the USA resulted in her resistance to having any further dealings with them:

> The hospice call here periodically wanting to know if they can help us with bereavement, and ... I know it's not right, but I would, one of these days love to just say, "You know, you didn't help me before, how're you gonna help me now?". So that sour grapes is not gonna help, but we found our own support systems.
> (Laura)

Laura also rejected the notion of pre-bereavement counselling and preparation for death as she said: 'that's like throwing in the towel to me. If my son refused to accept that he was dying, I was right along with him ... I was going with a miracle'. This suggests that before professionals attempt any pre-bereavement preparation, there needs to be an understanding of the readiness or otherwise of the family who may be distressed by such an approach.

In contrast, Bianca's story tells us how ill-prepared she and her husband Ryan were for his death and how, unlike Ian's mother, she felt she would have benefited from pre-bereavement counselling. We saw earlier in this chapter how Bianca was unable to internalise the reality of her husband Ryan's impending death. She told me how this 'lack of preparation' affected her bereavement:

> Because Ryan and I hadn't really spoken about his death, no one had sat with us and really helped us to plan ... what he would want for a funeral, what he would want to do with his stuff when he died. I struggled so much because it was suddenly my responsibility. I couldn't understand how he was gone ... I couldn't understand that he was dead ... I went back to see her [the Nurse Consultant] and the doctor a couple of times because I was extremely distressed about what had happened, and I couldn't understand how he'd died or why he'd died ... They maybe had to explain it two or three times to me ... what had happened, because I just ... I wasn't in the right place. I couldn't understand how it had happened and why it had happened ... and I was also linked up to the psychiatric services afterwards because ... I started to self-harm because ... I couldn't deal with what had happened ... I was really confused, and I just couldn't believe that he'd gone ... If I had to do it again, I would want someone there that was specifically trained, you know, dealing with young people and saying, you know, "He is gonna die, and you and I are gonna spend an hour a week, or whatever, preparing for this, and I'm gonna talk you through what happens ... I'm gonna talk you through the emotion you're gonna feel afterwards so you know that it's okay, so that you don't suddenly start ..." you know I was cutting myself, I was drinking ... all sorts of things just to numb the pain out ... because I was so confused, and I just didn't, I didn't know what was going on was okay, and I thought I was losing the plot. I didn't know what grief and bereavement was ...
> (Bianca)

The intensity of Bianca's grief and the unimaginable loss in becoming a widow at the age of 20, precipitated a crisis through which she was supported by psychiatric services. Could this crisis have been averted if she had received a different kind of support around the time of Ryan's death? This is, of course, an unanswerable question, but unlike Laura she believed she would have benefited from it.

One of the post-bereavement problems for parents and families is that during the final stages of the young person's life there will be a great deal of activity, many comings and goings in the home, and attention from professionals. Although this period is of course stressful and exhausting, it carries the family through on a momentum created by the intense commotion. When such activity stops abruptly after the death, the loss can be exacerbated by suddenly feeling alone and abandoned, which can throw family relationships into crisis as each member of the family deals with the loss, perhaps unable to support the other members of the family. This can be the case for the parents of children with long-term chronic conditions, and of the TYAs with cancer. Clare addressed the issue as follows: 'You'd gone from like really ... I don't know ... a manic, you know, in and out ... people in ... and it was just so quiet here'. But, like the mother who said counselling had opened 'a can of worms', Clare did not want counselling as she found it difficult to talk about Joe's death. Interestingly, she said she did not mind talking to me about it – perhaps because I hadn't known him – but that she would find it difficult to see the professionals who had cared for him to allow them to offer her support as: 'it'd be really hard to see [them] because it was just too close':

> We haven't [had counselling] ... I don't really want to ... I find it difficult talking to people that don't know. I mean I'll talk to you but ... that didn't know Joe, do you know what I mean? So to sort of sit and ... you know ... when they talk about counselling and things like that, I just think: "Well, you don't know ..."
> (Clare)

It was also clear from Clare's account that the impact on siblings can be lasting and profound. Members of the family dealt with Joe's illness and death differently, and this seemed to her son Jed to be a sign that the family was 'breaking apart':

> I don't think that he [surviving son Jed] liked the way that it was ... he didn't like the family being broken ... His fear, all the way through when Joe was ill, was: the whole family's going to break up and everyone's going to go their own ways – and everyone was all battling against each other because we was all ... you know ... with Joe's illness ... I dealt with it one way, Gary dealt with it another way and we was all battling against each other and he didn't know ... he didn't like that. He wanted it to be as it had always been, and it wasn't, because it just wasn't possible to be that way anymore. And that was his big fear, is that everything was going to fall apart. And I think now he realises that he doesn't want it to fall apart, so he wants to be ... he wants to have a family, I think. And that's ... you know it's never going to be the same. It never will be the same. There's nothing ... you know, nothing's going to be the same again, it never will, you know.
> (Clare)

This account might suggest that some support from an external source would have been welcomed, yet Clare expressed considerable ambivalence about the prospect of counselling. Even though she also said how 'quiet' the house became once Joe had died and all the professionals disappeared, she appeared not to want continued contact with the staff who had cared for Joe. In contrast, Karen's account shows how differently families may manifest their needs after the death, she expressed considerable anger at having been 'abandoned' by those who had cared for her son Mason:

> I wasn't very happy with the way certain things were dealt that way at all. And I did write a letter after Mason died to ... Mason's consultant, and said I felt that we'd put his life in their hands for two and a half years and then the day they told us there was no more they could do for him, we walked out of that hospital and we never heard from them again ... Apparently that letter has gone very, very far and wide. I've had an apology from [the consultant] over the phone; I've had apologies from [the nurse consultant] and it has taught them that they need to have an end of life team.
> (Karen)

It is clear from Karen's comment that, having established what she believed to be a meaningful relationship with the staff caring for her son, she expected this would extend to the period after he was discharged when his condition became untreatable. Beckie, whose daughter Billie had died on the same unit as Mason, gave a similar account:

> I have to say, I felt completely and utterly dumped by [the unit]. As soon as we left, that was it. There's nothing. It's just nothing. It's like we never existed. And I spent ... you know, I spent more time with those people than I did with my own family. I mean, I don't mean on a personal level I was dumped, I mean ... we just ...didn't exist anymore, because our child was dying, or our child was dead. She wasn't a patient anymore, so therefore nothing ... That was my "home", you know ...over 2 years, that's where I lived. I spent more time there than I did at home. You know, I saw the nurses more than I saw my husband. And then suddenly, that's it, they're out of your life, there's nothing. I didn't know anything about any support groups or anything that went on at [the hospital]. I wasn't contacted by anybody.
> (Beckie)

The extended times spent on the ward and lengthy period during which parents may come to regard the hospital as their 'second home' result in the sudden termination of contact feeling like abandonment. If this cessation of contact is followed swiftly by the death of the child, the parents can feel the lack of subsequent interest or engagement from the health professionals as very painful – it is as if it negates the regard in which they felt their child, and the value of his or her life, was held. Although both Karen and Beckie eventually became members of the bereavement group set up by the unit in which their children had died, it came late for them. They needed something more immediate to act as an intervention at the point of loss and death, to mitigate the feelings of abandonment.

Of course hospitals are primarily places of treatment, and a bed vacated at discharge or by a death will be filled by the next patient requiring the attention and care of the staff. Although at one level this is understood by parents, the bond they feel they have developed with staff is difficult to sever. However, hospitals are not as well equipped or prepared as hospices to offer bereavement support, particularly as this may be needed not only for a few months after the death, but possibly for several years, as Sarah clarifies:

> The children's hospice movement are excellent at supporting the family after the death of a child, as are the adult hospice movement [but] ... not in a hospital setting ... I think it's much harder for the hospitals. So if the young adults die on a hospital ward, which often happens at the moment ... there isn't the support within the hospital environment to offer bereavement support. And families often need that for 2 or 3 years after the death of their young person. It's a long time to be offering that support.
> (Sarah)

Whether or not the hospital where the death took place can offer ongoing support, the place where their son or daughter died continues to be of great significance to bereaved parents. For Pam and her husband Nick, the place where Amy died remained meaningful. In memory of their daughter, Pam and Nick had set up the 'Amy Food Campaign' to provide tasty, tempting food from a vending machine in the unit's kitchen. The machine was sponsored by a major supermarket, which agreed to keep it stocked with chilled food for a year. During the interview she told me the about their importance of continued involvement with both the location and the people through the campaign:

The 'Amy Food Campaign'
And one of the nicest things that happened at the unit is, when we had Amy's funeral we asked for donations and we actually got a lot of money. And we wanted all the money to go to the unit. And so we thought what we would like the money spent on and we chatted with the play specialist on the unit. And so you know, we decided ... what we wanted the money spent on ... we actually bought some of the things ourselves, and some of the things the unit bought. And so one particular day we'd arranged with the unit that we would go up and take these things up that we had bought – and this was 4 months after we lost Amy. And so, obviously, going back to the unit was very, very hard. But we just felt it was something we had to do. But do you know, they'd made a little tea party for us in the kitchen and so many people were told that we were coming, and so many people came in to see us. And we just felt so proud to think that Amy had meant so much to all those people, that they wanted to come and see us and in their way pay their respects. Because when you think how many

families they see on that ward, in that unit, and how many children I know that they do lose, and yet they still found the time to do that for us. Amy's consultants came in to see us, the nurses, the play specialists, administrators [and other] staff. We were just so proud. So, you know, the support that we've had from the unit has been unbelievable.

And since then we have actually been back four times, I think, now: once for the launch of the food campaign. And then the other times we've taken things that we've bought for the ward. And we're going up again just before Christmas with a selection of hats for the patients ... We just feel like we're coming home in a way, because we were there for 6 months, on the ward, and all the doctors and the nurses, they became like an extended family to us. And the fact that it's where Amy died, when we get to the hospital we go straight to the front door – have you seen a very large stone out the front? Well every time we went Amy always sat on that stone, because she loved stones and crystals and she couldn't get over the size of it. Every time we went she sat on that stone. And when we go now, we have to go and sit on it for her. And we just feel so close to her when we're up there. I can't explain it to people. You know people have said to us, "Why do you want to go back there?", and they can't understand it. But we just find it so meaningful to do it.

(Pam)

It is clear that the place where Amy died continues to hold significant meaning for her parents – indeed, it is almost like a shrine to them; should the stone ever be moved or replaced, it seems likely that it would be distressing for Pam and Nick, yet would the hospital administration ever consider such a possibility? The sense of violation felt by parents whose son had died in a hospital that was subsequently demolished was expressed by Steve, who told me how hard it had been to witness the destruction of the place where his son lost his life:

We walked round it last time we was up here. And it's the first time we'd actually walked round it since they knocked it down. I mean, the chapel's still there because that's listed. But what I didn't realise is – I don't know if you realise this? – but the wall that fronted the teenage ward, which was actually the side of the hospice wall, is actually still there. It's still intact. Just that wall. If you look from that side, it's all there. You go round the other side, there's nothing. There's just the wall standing there. He actually died in that ward ... on 29 September 2004.

(Steve)

The significance of the part of the wall that remained may seem surprising, but Steve talked of it, as Pam talked about the stone, as though it were a place of pilgrimage, a place to be close to his lost son, which had been desecrated by wanton destruction. Both Pam and Steve were members of the bereavement group I attended, and it is to the role of such groups that we now turn.

The role of bereavement support groups

We have seen how bereavement support can play a vital role for parents and families for some time after the death of their son or daughter, and this support can be offered in a variety of ways. One model is that of the bereavement support group where family members meet to discuss how their loss is affecting them, and to share stories and feelings with each other:

> I think the bereavement support groups are very important, because I've lost a lot of young adults over the past year and, talking to the parents, they will all say that if they happen to read something – and perhaps it's a mum worried that somebody else is feeling the same feelings as she is, or happen to have a similar sort of day – that's an incredible support, just to know that somebody else is going through a similar experience to you, and actually you're not going mad or you're not completely losing it ... because parents understand other parents far better than we can. And I think that's very supportive. I think sometimes it's easier for mums ... A lot of the dads are not great talkers, and they find that support and that group work difficult.
> (Sarah)

However, Sarah went on to say she did not think it was wise to put a group of parents together without a facilitator as there was a danger that while everyone talked about their experiences the group would not be able help people to move on. A facilitator might be a social worker, counsellor or family therapist organised through the hospice movement.

Despite Sarah's recognition that hospitals may find it harder to offer bereavement support, I was invited to attend a bereavement support group facilitated by a nurse consultant from a hospital-based TCT Unit. The group had been established as a result not only of understanding that bereaved families may be in need of continuing support, but also from the realisation that bereaved parents may form an attachment to those who treated and tried to save their child's life. Indeed, some parents felt that only a professional, who had known their child intimately and cared for them throughout their illness, could understand the loss.

In the group meeting I attended, parents used the forum in various ways: some were vociferous, tearful, expressed anger and sought to find meaning in the loss, whereas others simply listened. Pam, who agreed to be interviewed by me after the session, attended with her husband but said relatively little during the group. However, during my subsequent interview with her she said:

> Well it's something that I don't talk about ... in fact I don't even think I've said these things to anybody. And, maybe in a way, it might be good for me to be able to talk about it. So thank you for giving me the opportunity ... Obviously, you realise that I'm upset and I suppose I go to the groups and I just sort of listen ... I know that if I started to talk about it, I would just get so upset – and I suppose because I don't know a lot of the people there well enough, why I probably have never mentioned it. But maybe one day I will, I don't know.
> (Pam)

The group's discussion covered a wide range of issues and topics including: the significance of birthdays and anniversaries – how they were remembered and how the day was spent; speculation about what their lost son or daughter would be doing if they had lived; how important it was that their son's or daughter's friends remembered the day and kept in contact; the difficulty of accepting that other people's lives move on, and that their memory of significant dates may fade; the gap in the midst of the family; the 'empty chair' – being unable to eat at the table because of the missing child; the challenge of Christmas; the impact on the siblings; meaningful relics such as ashes – how and where they are kept and the importance of always having them nearby – and other people being 'spooked' by this; the care of the grave; the building of a 'shrine'; keeping hospital mementos, such as identity bracelets, medical notes and 'the sticky bits that go with Hickman lines'; what to do with their dead son's or daughter's clothes and other belongings; the loathing of medical environments; the traumatic nature of the experience they had all shared; guilt; resentment over tedious family and social demands that seem pointless and for which there is little energy; problems with form-filling; and the need to keep going because their son or daughter would be so annoyed if they gave into grief and stopped 'living'.

The bereavement group lasted for several hours and, as can be seen, the discussion ranged across a number of different topics, but interestingly no one talked about whether or not they had discussed their son's or daughter's death with them, despite the literature suggesting that this can be crucial to the bereavement process. Nevertheless, whatever the topic under discussion, there was clearly an immediate understanding from all the group members of exactly what others were talking about. It is impossible to do justice to the transcript of this group, which runs to 86 pages, but the extract below gives a privileged glimpse not only of a selected topic but also of the intimacy of the interaction between group members. The topic I have chosen, facilitated by Vikky, is 'what to do with the ashes':

Beckie: She's got her own alcove. We got it built in when we got the extension done.

Joan: Ahh, in the alcove, how nice.

Beckie: She just fits in nicely there. All her bits ... yes. The workmen thought we were a bit mental but ...

Joan: Yes. Yes, I get that very strange look, because our television broke and because Stuie's by the telly ... and when the guys came I said to Phillip ... I wasn't there, and I said to Phillip, "Did you move Stuie?" and he went, "The bloke was going ..." He was unbolting the TV and he kept looking down, he said, "And I just went, oh I'll just move my son" and he went, "Okay".

Vikky: Did [you] actually say that to the TV man?

Joan: Yes. And because he came yesterday, sort of yesterday, to put the telly back ... oh no, Friday ... And I was there, and I'd moved him because I thought it was a bit hard for them really, you know. I did think ...

Beckie: I was like that when the builders came in, because of all the dust. I don't like dust anyway, so I was walking around with Billie like this. We were running upstairs with her when it got too much ...

Joan: Yes. And I did move him when the TV ... but I put him on the side next to his photograph. I didn't move him out the room or anything. But Phillip said to me that, you know, "If we have friends round for a meal do you think it's ...?". Like he finds it a bit more difficult now, when other people are there. And I said, "If it's close friends I don't, because they know anyway and they were all there when he died". So I don't have a problem with that. But you know, other people are a bit ... it's just the eyes, you see them, and they sort of go ... You know, first of all I think they probably think it's an animal; they don't really think it's actually a person in that little box.

Pam: Perhaps they think he's going to pop out ...

Pam: Well, we took Amy with us to France. She's been to France twice, through the tunnel. [laughter]

Pam: Strapped in with the seatbelt.

Joan: Yes, we have Stuie in the back of the car with the dog when we go to Devon. It freaks a few people out, but ... his sort of seatbelt on him so he doesn't slip off the seat.

Pam: I just hope we don't get stopped at customs. We got pulled over last time didn't we ...

Nick: We did but they never worried.

Vikky: Were you speeding? [laughter]

Pam: No, at the tunnel, they pulled us over didn't they ...

Nick: You know, just have a check – but nothing ...

Pam: But they thought the thing inside ... but they didn't ask to look in the box so that was fine.

Joan: And I suppose you'd have to have your certificate, wouldn't you?

Beckie: Would you? I don't know even know where that is.

Joan: I don't know.

Pam: No, I don't know.

Nick: I don't know.

Joan: I don't know what they would do. I hadn't even thought about it really.

Pam: No.

Joan: Mind you I haven't tried to get him on an aeroplane yet.

Pam: No.

Beckie: You can't open Billie's bag anyway because it's all ...

Joan: No, Stuart's one's all sealed.

Beckie: She's in a ... hers is about this big and it's silver and pink. And I used to think, "Oh, what if somebody breaks in and thinks it's valuable?".

[Interruption – mobile phone rings]

Steve: There's always one, isn't there.

Beckie: Yes ...

Joan: Well, we thought about having him made into a diamond, and then my friend said to me, "What would you do if you lost it?".

Beckie: Yes, that's crossed my mind. My friend's had some lovely glass jewellery made, but they only use a little bit and then ... and they use ... they make the glass and they use a bit of the glass to make the pendant, and then you can keep some of the glass in case something happens to that pendant. But I don't like the idea of splitting Billie's ashes up at all.

Pam: No.

Joan: No.

Nick: No.

Joan: See, Phillip thought it would be good – we could like take him places where we've been and everything. I just said, "Oh I'm not being funny, but I'm not opening it". I don't think ...

Beckie: I just don't like the idea of her being all over the place.

Joan: No.

Beckie: I don't know why.

Joan: No. But apparently the undertaker down the road said to me, that they can do it for us; they can send the ... I said, "But I'd want to follow that little bag wherever it was going".[laughter]

Beckie: Yes, you would.

Joan: Yes, that's actually it, I'd be a bit ... because it could come back different colours. So if it came blue, he didn't have blue eyes ...

I have left this 'script' largely unedited as I believe it shows how the group's participants bounced off each other, entering territory that would be risky for anyone not in their position who did not truly comprehend their loss. This was not a focus group set up for my benefit as a researcher, but a regular bereavement group of parents and one sibling, who all knew each other and had extended a generous invitation to me to observe. I asked no questions and did not contribute, so the exchanges in this extract are spontaneous and demonstrate profundity, banality, humour, empathy and respect – and perhaps most importantly, the unspoken knowledge that their shared loss binds them together across any social divides and is more significant than that which separates them. Later in the conversation about the significance of the ashes and the problem other people may have in understanding their meaning, Val says: 'It's just that most people haven't gone through the experience that we have of having their child die' .This comment makes explicit the subtext throughout, which assumes that other people, whether the builder, the TV repair man, the dinner guest or the customs officer, would simply not understand.

During the course of my interviews in the region these parents came from, it became apparent to me that not all those who might have benefited from the group were 'aware' of its existence. I asked Chris, 6 months after her son Ben died, whether she had received any support since Ben's death:

> We had a letter through, I think about 2 months after Ben died, saying there was ... a counselling support group for people that have died on the unit. I never took that up actually, no. To be honest, I think the first couple of months after your child's died you're quite numb. Everything's quite unbelievable and you're in a sort of a dream – you're in a daze. You don't really deal with things. I did go to see a counsellor three times, but just felt like there was nothing they could do for me. I was a mum grieving and I know it's time that will heal, and nothing else.
> (Chris)

However, when I told Chris about the bereavement group the TCT unit facilitated, she said:

> I just feel like a parent's grief is so different. To lose a child shouldn't happen. You shouldn't be burying your children. And I think it would be nice to talk to other parents that have lost children, just to feel that connection with them because ... I didn't know [about that group]. No, I didn't know.
> (Chris)

Sarah, the health professional who was present at the interview, also said she had been unaware of this bereavement support group. It may seem surprising that in the same discussion Chris said she had been told of a 'counselling support group', had chosen not to attend, but when I told her about the bereavement group she expressed an interest in talking to the parents who had been through the same experience. It is difficult to tell if she rejected the invitation to what was apparently the same bereavement group because the invitation came too soon when – as she says she was 'quite numb' – or because of the terminology that had been used.

Although the invitation to join this group may have been too early for Chris, other parents spoke of being left alone to manage their grief for too long. This suggests that each bereaved family and individual members of that family may need the support of such an intervention at different stages after their loss. Some may feel abandoned if the contact is left 'too long'; whereas others may not 'hear' what is being offered if it comes 'too soon'. This presents a problem for professionals offering help, suggesting that contact should be made early but, even if it is rejected initially, later attempts should be made to offer support. The models of grief in operation may suggest a linear progression through the process and propose a period of time taken to progress through each stage, but as we have seen, reactions to the loss of a child do not necessarily follow a predictable pattern – this does not mean the grief is 'dysfunctional', but it might be considered 'complicated' and require a flexible approach.

Although the discussion thus far has been primarily about parents' bereavement needs, it is also important to remember that at the older end of the adolescent/young adult age group the young person who dies may, like Bianca and Ryan, have been married and left behind a widowed partner. However, we can see from Bianca's account below that joining an inappropriate bereavement support group was unhelpful:

> I know that there's lots of services for mums and dads and brothers and sisters who've lost someone ... but being 20 and losing your husband ... I went to a support group once after he'd died, that someone had put me in touch with, and I was the youngest person in the room by about 40 years ... And walking into that room was horrific because people were just, like, "Who are you, and why are you here?". And having to tell them all, and they'd all had these amazing lives together and could share all these memories ... and I couldn't relate to any of them. There was no one that had understood the life experience that I'd just had ... I'd had 6 weeks, whereas they'd had, you know, 40-odd years ...and it just ... it seemed really unfair.
> (Bianca)

This bereavement group was clearly completely unsuitable for Bianca, and may have done more harm than good in that it made her loss seem even more 'unfair'. Bianca suggested that a support group for young people who had been widowed or lost their partner could be put in place for other young people in her position.

The children and young people, the impact of whose loss is the focus of this chapter, have died from a variety of illnesses: some of the deaths were predictable after lifelong chronic illness, whereas others were the result of an unexpected and acute illness. Runswick-Cole (2010: 813) points out there is a fallacy assumed by some: 'the death of a disabled child has sometimes been judged as being less important than the deaths of non-disabled children'. I asked Sheila, experienced in supporting bereaved parents of both children who had died from lifelong conditions and of adolescents who had died from a sudden and acute illness such as cancer, if she could discern any qualitative difference in how the loss in these very different circumstances affected parents' grieving. She said:

> I think the loss and the impact is exactly the same. I think that sometimes the treatment options ... can have different memories and different challenges for parents. But I think, when you meet together in a group, it's actually the impact of the loss is the same ... The impact of the loss is the same, but the losses can be very different, because obviously if it's things like they've maybe just "babbled" a little bit and then lost that, whereas if they've [been] diagnosed in adolescence your hopes and dreams would have been very different to a mother who knew that their child was maybe never going to achieve even reading. So I think the components of the loss are very different, but the impact of the loss is the same ... Everybody is very different ... but in the groups it doesn't seem to be very different for families, dependent on what the child dies from ... So we would run the group for a year and the parents would come for a year. So it would be whatever the diagnosis were of the children who'd died in that time-frame that you were taking the parents from ... And they're all very generous [to] each other, actually. It's very interesting that the oncology parents would maybe say, "But I had a child who was achieving", and the others would say, "But then you've lost what your child achieved".
> (Sheila)

Interestingly, Sheila points out that to lose a child under any circumstances – whether from a complex lifelong illness or an unexpected malignancy – the impact is very similar, and thus parents from both cohorts are included in the same bereavement support group and as she says are 'very generous' to each other, recognising the significance of the loss under different circumstances. Once again, we have returned to the deeply embedded notion in contemporary Western society that in any circumstances for children to pre-decease their parents is unnatural and unacceptable.

Discussion

Much of the discussion in this chapter could be applied to the preparation for the end of life and the bereavement needs of people in other circumstances – so which aspects of the accounts in this chapter relate particularly to the loss of a child? First, the strong sense that the death of a child before its parents is unacceptable can lead to parents being unwilling to broach the issue with their son or daughter. This may be more problematic if the illness has been a long one – when does it feel appropriate to raise the subject of death? If the child has transitioned from childhood through to young adulthood, at what point do parents relinquish control of the information and decision making? Brannen et al. (1994) say it is difficult enough under 'normal' circumstances for parents to relinquish control over their children's health, and when the diagnosis is terminal, family dynamics can be thrown into crisis. This situation can also be difficult for professionals to read, as it may be unclear who knows what and how information is shared and decisions made. Because the legality of sharing information with a child or young person may differ from country to country, or even from state to state in a single country, this makes any generalisations on the rights of a young person problematic. However, although the law may vary between countries, it is clear that the emotional impact on parents and the difficulties of disclosure know no national boundaries.

A guide for GPs in the UK (ACT 2011c) designed to help in supporting the end of life care for children offers the following guidance:

> Open awareness is the ideal as it allows for fears and concerns to be voiced and addressed, for better care plans to be negotiated and agreed; and for the child and family to feel more in control. Often child, family and professionals are each in different awareness contexts, or stuck in 'mutual pretence', usually because the truth is too distressing or difficult to handle. Generally it is fine to allow everyone to reach open awareness in their own time, but where blocked communication risks increasing a child's suffering (e.g. where a child is isolated and anxious), or where events are proceeding so fast that communication is crucial to plan, prepare and adapt, then you may need to intervene.
> (ACT 2011: 14)

The literature clearly indicates that an open awareness context is the best way to prepare a child or young person for death, and that this can also act as a preparation for bereavement for the family. It is also apparent from the literature that these debates go back decades, yet throughout the accounts in this chapter we can see that the management of communications at the end of a child's life may still be loaded with disagreement, uncertainty and ambiguity. Parents' approaches ranged from concealing the truth or avoiding the issue through to full disclosure, and the accounts make the emotional difficulties of full disclosure very plain. Yet there appears to be an assumption on the part of professionals that even if the parents decide to conceal the prognosis from their son or daughter, somehow the young person 'knows' they are dying. This assumption has been demonstrated in some of the accounts, where the medical professional has insisted the young person is fully aware, whereas the parents have been equally convinced that they are not. McCallum, Byrne and Bruera (2000) suggest that a child as young as 3 may have a 'rudimentary' understanding that they are going to die even if they have not been told, and yet we have seen cases where young people a great deal older than this refuse to accept the likelihood of their impending death. Ryan described his prognosis as a 'crock of shit', and his conviction that he would beat the cancer left his widow Bianca totally unprepared for his death. Ryan and Bianca had been 'told' and thus 'knew' that he would not survive, and yet they also did not 'know'; as Bianca said: 'no one had sat with us and really helped us to plan'. She suggested it would have been necessary to have someone trained in speaking to people of her age to sit with her repeatedly for an hour a week to take her through the process and prepare her. Whether this would really have prepared Bianca is impossible to say, but from her account we can see that the phenomenon of 'knowing and not knowing' presents a challenge to both professionals and families in managing information and preparing for death. In other cases we have seen that professionals and parents can clash in their approach to open awareness, which can cause additional distress at a traumatic time.

Turkoski (2003: 83) suggests that a useful response to a parent blocking truthful disclosure might involve:

- a consultation with an appropriate ethics committee
- continued discussions with the parent – perhaps revealing the patient's wish to know
- approaching the parent's spiritual advisor
- acknowledging the parent's pain.

and concludes that:

> Communication, understanding and support are going to be necessary for everyone involved ... the dying patient, the mother who is facing the loss of her child, and the professional staff who are suffering painful "ethical dissonance".
> (Turkoski 2003: 83)

Yet there are additional difficulties in judging if and how to tell a very young child, or a child with cognitive impairments, that they will die. The issues here are different, cases will vary, family relationships and ways of communicating will also differ, as will the attitudes and assumptions of the professionals. As Alderson (1992) points out, parents affect a child's maturity – thus those whose parents believe them to be immature remain so. This tendency may be increased for parents whose son or daughter has had a lifelong illness and whose physical or intellectual vulnerability may lead parents, understandably, to be particularly protective. Thus, individual assessments of a child's capacity and competence need to be based not only on chronological age, or even on a medical condition that may affect their cognitive abilities, but also on the context in which the parents and child communicate.

It is also apparent that the events leading up to the death have an impact on the bereavement and the grieving process. If families are left feeling angry that their wishes were not respected, that their son or daughter was not treated in the 'right' place by people who understood both their medical and emotional needs, if they were given inappropriate information, if they lost 'control' of the dying process or were unprepared for the physical manifestations of the end of life, the ramifications can be severe and ongoing.

Wiener et al. (2008) suggest that an advance care planning document, such as the *Five Wishes*, which is recognised as a legal document in 40 states in the USA, may be a vehicle that can assist in approaching the very challenging concept of talking to a young person about their impending death. The results of their study show that adolescents and young people are open to and interested in discussing their end of life care, and that the use of such a document can foster discussion with family and health professionals. The document covers the following:

- The Person I Want to Make Care Decisions for Me When I Can't
- The Kind of Medical Treatment I Want or Don't Want
- How Comfortable I Want to Be
- How I Want People to Treat Me
- What I Want My Loved Ones to Know.

(Wiener et al. 2008: 1310)

Preparation for bereavement is important, but so, too, is bereavement support after the death. Here, too, we see that there can be a discrepancy between what the families need and when they need it, and the assumptions made by professionals about what might be appropriate. Some families felt abandoned by their son's or daughter's health care professionals, others wanted no more to do with them. Some parents craved support, whereas others feared it would 'open a can of worms'. The period of time after the death when support was needed also varied between bereaved family members. We can see from Macdonald et al.'s study(2005) that returning to the hospital where their child died can be very difficult for parents, yet we have also seen in the interview data, the significance 'place' can assume and the feelings of violation that can result if it is demolished or even altered. These discrepancies suggest that the adoption of a single model of grief is unlikely to address the requirements of all those in need of bereavement support and that individualised approaches are necessary.

Parents indicated that some of the feelings of abandonment could be mitigated by the presence of staff at their child's funeral, but some professionals were unsure if this would be welcomed, whereas others said they would have to take annual leave and could therefore not afford regularly to attend the funerals of dead patients. Hospices were more likely than hospitals to provide time off to attend funerals, as this is seen as an element of the wider support offered by hospice services.

Not all bereaved family members want to belong to a formalised group, and may instead find other ways to manage their grief and remember their children; going to a memorial service, fund-raising, taking part in charitable events or undertaking voluntary work for the hospice or hospital where their child has died, can all be ways of dealing with the loss and maintaining a meaningful connection with a significant place and key people. However, it may be easier to undertake such activity if the care setting was a hospice rather than a busy city centre hospital far from home and with less chance of ongoing personal contact.

Lessons for best practice

The accounts from both family members and professionals indicate that the events leading up to the death of a son or daughter, and the support needed after the death, are not always well managed and understood. This appears to be related to a lack of communication, and uncertainty for families about what they can reasonably expect, and for professionals about what families want. The following points may be useful when professionals are faced with such a situation:

- Early interventions may be helpful to support families in discussing death with their son or daughter.
- Such pre-bereavement support may be helpful but must be approached with care at a point when the family has accepted that a cure will not take place.
- Only a limited understanding of a young person's capacity to deal with such information can be gleaned from their chronological age.
- Where there is disagreement about the appropriate way to communicate information about death, sensitive negotiation is required, perhaps involving specialist bereavement counsellors rather than relying on medical personnel.
- No assumptions should be made about how and when bereavement support will be needed – families can feel abandoned if they have been left for what they perceive to be 'too long', even if that period conforms to that suggested as appropriate by a model of grief.
- Support may be needed by siblings and grandparents as well as parents.
- The presence of professionals at a funeral is usually welcomed and taken as a tribute to the lost child.

Chapter 6
The Implications for Policy and Practice

Access to services

The provision of palliative and end of life care for children and young people is now an issue very much on the agenda; however, the empirical data in this book indicate that although policy documents on the provision of palliative and end of life care abound, there is considerable patchiness in provision and quality. Although a booklet published by CLIC Sargent (2006) suggests that families have choices about where their child will die, in reality these choices may be constrained by local provision and become merely 'alternatives' that may or may not be available. Many accounts in this book testify to parents struggling to find appropriate care in their preferred setting, which is reiterated by Liz, Head of Care at a hospice, who confirmed that a 'postcode lottery' may govern what resources are available to a child or young person at the end of their life:

> We try to be as fair as possible. It doesn't necessarily mean that two people with the same condition will automatically get the same allocation, because there's a huge postcode lottery. So somebody can have their needs assessed in one PCT (primary care trust) as... meaning that they should get a certain care package, and yet somebody with very, very similar needs, very similar family situation, in a different PCT... will be assessed completely differently.
> (Liz)

Liz continued by questioning whether the establishment of yet more children's hospices was the answer to this problem, commenting that raising money for a new children's hospice is what 'what people want to do when their child has died... it's part of the legacy'. However, she added, people do not want to fund the nurses and the carers who work there, so it is an unsustainable strategy and not necessarily the best use of resources. As well as the patchiness of provision referred to by Liz, gaps in services also affect the 16-18-year age group - again subject to a 'postcode lottery'. This can be a particular problem

Palliative and End of Life Care for Children and Young People: Home, Hospice and Hospital, First Edition. Anne Grinyer.
© 2012 John Wiley & Sons, Ltd. Published 2012 by John Wiley & Sons, Ltd.

for the young person with acute illness who has no history of care in their local community. Inventive local solutions can be found: for example, Saul, the Director of Day and Out Patient Services at an adult hospice, talked about how local paediatric services knew they should discharge their patients at the age of 16, but knowing that no one would pick them up they: 'jolly well ignore it – and hurrah to them'. This can, however, lead to teenagers outgrowing a service that may be perceived as 'hanging on' to them inappropriately and is not a long-term solution. In response to the 'care gap' Saul makes sure that his team, as the local specialist palliative care provider of an adult service, registers a member of the family – perhaps the mother – as being in need of care, thus finding a way to support the patient who has fallen between services.

We saw similar examples throughout the book of exceptions being made in both hospice- and community-based services, and even in some cases the compassion of individual professionals extending their care beyond their remit by stepping in to fill a gap in provision. For the parents of a young person in need of pain relief at the end of their life, the additional distress caused by struggling to find appropriate services is almost unendurable and their gratitude to those who 'bend the rules' is immense. Yet provision should not be reliant on goodwill and compassion, rather care and support should be provided as part of a seamless service embracing all ages and geographical locations.

There appears to be enough evidence in this book from both families and professionals to suggest that there is a need for provision to be regulated – at the highest level – so that wherever a child, young person or their family live they will be entitled to appropriate services. Perhaps unsurprisingly, provision is regarded as a local problem; there is little understanding of how challenges are experienced in other regions or by other services, apparently no national overview of provision and no automatic streamlining of transition between services. Yet there is also evidence that where cooperation and collaboration have been established, services can work well together, and transition from one service to another can be achieved seamlessly.

Access to appropriate services can be related directly to how well liaison and communication is managed, but where boundaries exist and relationships have not been developed in advance, communication can be problematic. As can be seen in the later section of this chapter on 'best practice', some Teenage Cancer Trust (TCT) units have developed excellent relationships with other care providers. However, for other TCT units effective communication with services can be complex. For example, care providers in rural areas may be a considerable distance away, in some cases across mountainous terrain, whereas equal difficulty might be experienced in urban conurbations that can cover multiple PCTs and district general hospitals (DGHs). These services may also have different policy and resource issues of their own, in terms of hospice provision alone one respondent to the 2009 Service Evaluation said: 'We have over 10 hospices adult and children's available to us in our catchment area some children's hospices take up to 19-year-olds others don't'; thus, the seamless transfer of patients at the end of their life can be problematic. As Zephyrine Barbarachild, who undertook the TCT service evaluation in 2011, observed:

The TCT units vary considerably, depending on their location (urban/rural/semi-rural) and the areas they cover. Urban-based units, which serve large areas, which potentially profoundly affect the outcomes for TYAs (teenagers and young adults), are mitigated by the communications skills of individuals in positions of influence and/or the willingness of partners to cooperate and collaborate on the primary concern: enabling TYAs and their families to experience the best death possible.
(Zephyrine Barbarachild)

The TCT units provide an exemplar, but the situation for children with other illnesses may not in effect be very different. For the children with complex life-limiting conditions, there needs to be effective communication between their hospice carers, the general practitioner (GP) and hospital services. Where this works well it can streamline the provision of care, but again, potentially, with multiple services across a wide geographical area, relationships can be difficult to establish. If, in addition, there is uncertainty about who should provide the care, parents can find themselves caught in a breakdown of communication between services.

Transition from paediatric to adult services

The challenges to both staff and patients providing age-appropriate care to TYAs with cancer have been increasingly recognised in policy documents (e.g. Association of Children's Palliative Care 2007; DH 2008; Marsh et al. 2011), clinical texts (e.g. Arbuckle et al. 2005, Kelly and Gibson 2008) and academic writing (e.g. Grinyer and Thomas 2004; Grinyer 2007a). We have seen attempts by adult hospices to extend their provision to a younger age group and by paediatric hospices to extend their provision to an older age group – but the extension of provision for TYAs does not come without difficulties. The challenges lie not only in appealing to TYAs, but also in integrating them with the core users and staff unused to the age group.

Yet the difficulties of integrating TYAs into hospice services is not limited to those with acute illness diagnosed in their teenage years. The testimonies in this book illustrate how transition is also a difficult time for those young people who have been born with a life-limiting condition. Although they may be familiar with the care setting in a children's hospice, when they reach their teens many will find the provision no longer offers them the social support they need, or an age-appropriate environment and their separation from 'normal' teenage activities is exacerbated by being cared for in close proximity to infants and children.

This clearly presents a problem for care providers – there are very few adolescent hospices and the likelihood of many more being built is not great. However, age-appropriate care does not need to depend only on a dedicated age-specific care setting but can be based on a philosophy of care, for which there is an effective and proven model as developed by the TCT Units.

Although some teenage cancer patients' issues may be disease-specific, other aspects of being a teenager with a life-threatening illness transcend the illness and are simply about being a teenager. There are training issues for staff who have not opted to care for this age group and who are more comfortable with either young children or older adults, but there are enough examples of the successful extension of care in non-age-specific settings to suggest that the model can be adopted and applied to a variety of services.

George and Hutton (2003) identify the ideals to which the approach to the management of dying teenagers should aspire, including the willingness to treat patients as equals, which, they argue, means being open and honest even if it runs counter to parents' wishes about disclosure. George and Hutton argue that although non-disclosure may be a short-term advantage, distress inevitably results from the patient imagining the worst rather than being able to enter into a truthful dialogue; they claim that the way to make the acceptance of the lost future for the young person as healthy as possible is to face the reality and engage with it. Yet we have seen the difficulties that both parents and young people may have in addressing end of life issues. Thus, immense care and sensitivity are necessary to avoid some of the distressing encounters related in this book, where the application of the accepted model of good practice (open awareness) has overridden an individual family's preferred way of managing this upsetting issue.

George and Hutton also say that despite death being inevitable, markers of achievement such as exams are important, as are any activities that foster socialisation and normality. Professionals also need to accept that they can-not make everything all right, and that crises and emotions are inevitable but can be used positively to move the patient forward. Teamwork is also vital, as is the interdisciplinary care needed for this age group and, as George and Hutton note, the disparate views of paediatric and adult care need to be overcome to enable both groups to make a valuable contribution to the child in transition.

Training and resource needs

Sheetz and Bowman (2008) address the training needs of doctors who are called on to communicate information relating to the impending death of children and young people. These authors suggest that the proportion of physicians at the children's medical centre in their study who felt competent to give difficult news to families is high at 74%, whereas their confidence in managing end of life symptoms is low at 23%. However, according to Sheetz and Bowman, few physicians are interested in obtaining additional training, and are more likely to refer their patients to a palliative care consultant, which, Sheetz and Bowman say, argues in favour of hospital-based palliative care teams and for specialty training in paediatric palliative care. We have also seen that the difficulty lies not only in giving bad news to families, but also in understanding the complexity of family dynamics and negotiating the sharing of information with the child or young person. This suggests that many professionals would benefit from training in these skills so that open awareness and models of good practice can be implemented in a manner that does not cause conflict between the family and professionals.

It became clear from the service evaluation of palliative and end of life care for TYAs with cancer (Grinyer and Barbarachild 2011), that there are several specialised training and resource needs associated with offering this care. Although there are pathway models designed for adults, there was nothing available specifically for TYAs, whose needs may be very different. Many participants expressed a need for an age-specific care pathway, and such a pathway would also be a helpful framework for the age group with other illnesses and lifelong conditions, which mean that their needs at the end of life as TYAs may not be met – as we have seen in the section on transition.

However, although the young people have specific needs, so also do the staff who care for them and a number of concerns were expressed about their need for support. Physical and emotional support were found to some extent to be provided between team members, but there was also a need for more formalised clinical support. Distress was experienced by staff when they were 'outside their comfort zone'. A distinction was made between supporting end of life care in an acute hospital setting and in hospices where staff are expert in this specialist field. Hospital staff who are confident in offering support during treatment do not necessarily feel they have the skills to do the same at the end of life, despite effectively fulfilling the same role as a hospice. This can apply to caring for children with all conditions and at all ages at the end of life, in a setting where the focus is on treatment.

Other staffing issues raised by the TCT service evaluation (2011) included the shortage of nurses, and a need was expressed for specialist staff to be available out of hours, as end of life care pain control and symptom management can be difficult for senior house officers because of their relative lack of experience. There was a concern in some settings that staff were becoming over-involved with the patients, which can be problematic. The need to keep developing and building skills was thought important and among the list of training needs identified in several settings was:

- training in palliative and end of life care advanced communication skills
- training in the assessment of needs
- training in pre-bereavement and bereavement counselling
- training in disease management and pain control
- training in group work facilitation skills
- training in teamwork dynamics
- training and awareness-raising with others: community networks, hospices
- service development training for working with hospices.
  (Grinyer and Barbarachild 2011: 18)

Skills required to support home deaths were also found wanting in some areas. The management of portacaths, Hickman lines and other technologies may be unfamiliar to some community-based nursing staff. Yet again, this can be dependent on local services and there is a strong argument to be made for staff caring for a child or young person at home being trained in such technologies. Yet one TCT nurse consultant, said that the advanced nature of palliative care as it is delivered in hospital is rarely addressed; this means that what can be delivered in an inpatient setting may be difficult to deliver in an outpatient setting or at home. For example, the use of an epidural for pain control might tie the young person to hospital, because community-based services are unlikely to be able to manage epidural pain relief. Thus, if complex symptom management is in place in hospital but cannot be delivered at home, it is necessary to be honest about this so that the young person and their family can decide in advance which is more important - the 'bottom line' may be a judgement between the preference for place of death and pain relief.

However, as the nurse consultant pointed out, there is no point putting a plan in place if it cannot be delivered, thus the basic infrastructure needs to be established well in advance of when it is actually needed. It may be, as this nurse consultant said, that it is not only important to establish goodwill, but also professionals in the many care settings involved may need to be willing to extend the boundary of their role to be able to deliver an appropriate service to a young person at the end of their life. This should not be dependent on one person but should be based on a team approach and, if this works, it should mean a parent is not forced to spend the last weeks or days of their son's or daughter's life trying to obtain appropriate care.

Best practice

Instances of best practice were found throughout the research and evaluation process, and the following examples are drawn from the whole range of care settings. However, they are not necessarily setting-specific and many can be implemented across different services for different age groups. For instance, a CLIC Sargent clinical psychologist in the TCT service evaluation said it is important to gauge how much input a family wants, and tailor input to their needs by letting them know support is available as, when and how they could benefit from it. This seems an eminently sensible way of interacting with families across a range of services - and it is perhaps surprising that it does not already happen routinely in all circumstances.

Throughout the fieldwork it became apparent that good relationships and close links between services can transform the experience for the patient and their family, and where effective communication has been successful the effect is described as 'more than the sum of its parts' with, for instance, in some units all clinicians sharing an electronic patient record. In the TCT service evaluation, to ensure good communication, a palliative care team (PCT) attended the multidisciplinary team (MDT) meetings and this was coupled with a reciprocal arrangement where the TCT team also attended PCT meetings. Continuous communication, integration and co-working with allied health care professionals are also important: physiotherapists, dieticians and occupational therapists can all help improve planning – especially at the end of life. The need for good communication was taken one step further by a TCT professional nursing lead, who discussed the possibility of reciprocal training through working with hospices on a training exchange – a mutual exchange should ensure that resource implications are minimal while at the same time delivering significant benefit for both parties. Where the children or young people are cared for outside an end of life care setting, involving the specialist palliative care service early in the process can help build relationships between them and patients, and alleviate the fear that can be associated with palliative care.

The role of MDTs cannot be overstated, particularly when managing end of life care for young people whose lives may be chaotic and problematic – far from the idealised scenario of well-behaved grateful patients living in the midst of a supportive family. The TCT service evaluation (Grinyer and Barbarachild 2011) provides evidence of the strategic importance of the role of the MDT. For example, at a weekly MDT video-conference with a local hospital, the meeting, chaired by the lead clinical nurse specialist, was attended by her community nursing service (CNS) colleague, the CLIC Sargent social worker, three consultants and two other doctors. The four cases discussed at some length illustrate the wide variety of patients including: a 16-year-old South African asylum-seeker, living in a children's unit, having been trafficked and being treated for hepatitis B and a liver tumour. Another patient under discussion was a young man of 23 referred for a bone marrow transplant, who continually failed to take his medication. He was described as 'leading a chaotic social life', which could compromise his post-transplant adherence, leaving him at risk of transplant-related mortality. In another instance, a TCT unit was required to care for a young person in homeless accommodation, which resulted in some concern about how best to support him at the end of his life. As a result, the CLIC Sargent clinical psychologist said: 'three clinical staff in the team put together an informal training package for the staff there [at the homeless hostel]' (Grinyer and Barbarachild 2011: 21). In such cases, the MDT may need to liaise not only with fellow health and social care professionals, but also with the police, probation services and immigration officers.

Although the children with complex life-limiting illnesses may not have had the same 'opportunity' for their lives to become chaotic, the impact on their families of caring for a disabled child may have resulted in the family struggling with, for example, increased stress, economic hardship, strained social relationships and social isolation (Woolfson 2004). Once again, this may necessitate liaison between a variety of services to ensure that the families are adequately supported to manage the death.

Outreach work can also be extended from a PTC to other hospitals in the region so, for example, clinical nurse specialists can advise staff in non-specialist settings. A TCT clinical nurse specialist identified additional ways that 24-hour support can contribute, by liaising with local services:

There's a multiprofessional operational policy on the hospital intranet, which I review and update every day. And we have the PATCH [24-hour telephone advice] service. We have 3 years' funding for this out-of-hours service, which gives phone advice to families and professionals, wherever the patient is. Once the medical decision has been made that a patient is no long curative, PATCH kicks in, and we arrange to meet with local services (Grinyer and Barbarachild 2011: 21).

The involvement of patients can also be empowering, as a CLIC Sargent social worker noted:

There's an ethos behind CLIC Sargent guidelines, which includes user participation. For example, there was a patient on the interview panel for the new social worker here. And CLIC Sargent send out questionnaires to families after treatment, for service-user feedback. (Grinyer and Barbarachild 2011: 21)

The underpinning philosophy of 'getting patients to where they want to be: physically, mentally and socially', includes enabling the young people to die where they want - a recurrent desire in the accounts in this book. Evidence from the TCT service evaluation (Grinyer and Barbarachild 2011) suggests that with the cooperation of a wide variety of professionals, including the ambulance service, pharmacists and district nurses, getting a patient home to die can be achieved in as little as 4 hours, demonstrating that collaboration and cooperation between services both within and outside the hospital makes the logistics possible. However, such a manoeuvre could only be successful with forward planning and if good relationships have already been established between the services. Once the patient has been discharged and is living at home, equipment is likely to be required; however, an occupational therapist from this study indicated that her role extended beyond arranging equipment such as stair-lifts or hoists, to include more personal support with activities such as writing, looking at photos and facilitating the opportunity to 'talk things through... even if there's no future' (Grinyer and Barbarachild 2011: 21).

Other suggestions for best practice included:

- successful transitioning to adult services
- the need for flexibility and sensitivity
- choice of place of death, and to feel supported with all relevant information
- a joint supportive MDT approach
- ensuring the family are offered support following an assessment of their needs
- to be both patient-centred and family-centred and to follow the individual's wishes as much as possible
- Recognise that a good death is not necessarily a textbook death
- a mortality/morbidity meeting (M&M) after the patient's death, which is minuted, recording what needs to change.
  (Grinyer and Barbarachild 2011: 22)

However, any model of best practice needs to be flexible because 'one size does not fit all'. Thus 'best practice' needs to be adaptable rather than consisting of a rigid set of guidelines – perhaps the term 'good practice', based on the 'principles' referred to above, would be the basis of a more useful way of thinking. This is reinforced by a response from the 2009 service evaluation:

> Our children's and young people's symptom care and outreach team will care for patients up to 25 years, and work collaboratively with local hospice community care teams, primary care services (children and adults) and the adult palliative care team... One size does not fit all in this case and to ensure a package of care that meets the needs of the patient and family takes a considerable amount of organizing and negotiation...especially as palliative care may take place over a prolonged time of period (up to a year in some cases), with changing physical/psychological/social support needs during that time, access to active therapy (chemotherapy, radiotherapy and phase I&II clinical trials) may be needed too. There are examples of very good care and examples of not so good care. What makes it work is proactive clinical leadership, patient involvement and good teamwork rather than a single model of care.

The final sentence in the quote above may be crucial and is worth reiterating as it captures the need for *adaptability, organisation, leadership, teamwork and patient involvement* in a situation that may be changing over the course of a significant period of time. It may also be tempting to assume that the patient has a family; but, as we have seen from the previous examples, to draw up guidelines based on such a premise would be inadequate under some circumstances. Thus, the 'guiding principles' approach would have greater applicability in cases where a young person does not belong to a traditional nuclear family or has social problems in addition to their illness.

Although the examples of good practice discussed so far relate to the palliative and end of life care phase, after the death of the young person the family still needs support. There is evidence throughout this book that the place where their son or daughter was cared for remains significant, as does continued contact with the staff who remember them. It can be helpful to offer ongoing bereavement support, as and when individual family members need it, and an assurance that contact can be maintained. Even if it is not taken up, the knowledge that it is available and that bereaved families know that they have not been abandoned or forgotten can be important in its own right. It became clear from the bereavement group cited in the previous chapter that it is important that professionals listen to what parents and siblings want and need rather than decide on their behalf how a service should look. As this group's convenor said:

> One of the next things that we'll be looking at is bereavement support for siblings and what's necessary and what do we need to put in place... it's important, because otherwise, what will happen... health professionals

will go off in a little huddle and they'll decide how it should look... so it would be far more sensible to actually ask the young people themselves. (Vikky)

Although much of the discussion of 'best practice' has been drawn from that offered to TYAs with cancer, many of the same principles apply to children with other life-threatening and life-limiting conditions. The need for excellent communications between services; listening to what the parents and children want; taking into account their family circumstances; making sure that community-based staff have the expertise to administer pain relief and other interventions at home; planning in advance and being honest about what the different options for care can realistically offer; and continuation of support for the family after the death – all are applicable whatever the age of the child or the nature of their illness.

However, there are some key differences for the families of the children with life-limiting illness, who will have had a much longer relationship with the health professionals caring for their child. For the families of the children with complex life-limiting conditions, who may find themselves in receipt of services for which they are very grateful but to which they have very limited access, there may be ways for them to have more control over their access to support. For example, we have already seen that a parents' user group, a Facebook page for parents and a parent-run bereavement group can act to empower families. In addition, the provision of an 'eHealth' service can enable parents to feel they have greater access to support, advice, a wider community of users and choice about when they can access much-needed inpatient respite care (Grinyer, Payne and Barbarachild 2010). eHealth is a relatively recent term for health care practice, which is supported by electronic processes and communication. Meyer et al. (2010) argue that information technology has been shown to empower users in the management of chronic conditions, ameliorating the impact on individuals and families. Among its many benefits, Eysenbach (2001) suggests that eHealth encourages a new relationship between service users and health professionals, and enables decisions to be made in a shared manner.

Contrasts and commonalties between the needs of families in the two studies

Clearly, the two studies drawn on in this book – the evaluation of the needs of the parents and families of children with complex life-limiting conditions, and the research into palliative and end of life care for TYAs with cancer – raise a number of different and contrasting issues.

The perception of services may vary widely between the two groups. The parents of children with complex life-limiting conditions value inpatient respite care highest: although home-based care is, of course, integral to their ability to keep their child at home, the much-needed complete break for the family while their child is in hospice respite care allows batteries to be recharged and home-based care to resume with renewed energy. However, the families of the TYAs with cancer may view the difference between inpatient and home-based care very differently: they may prioritise the ability to access home-based care in order to achieve a home death. For some, inpatient care may represent a failure to provide a home death, because admission to a hospice or hospital can result in their son or daughter dying in that setting. Yet paradoxically, it seems to be the families of the TYAs who can find it most difficult to access home-based care – particularly if their son or daughter is aged between 16 and 18, whereas the parents of the children with life-limiting conditions may find access to inpatient care restricted and insufficient to meet their needs.

Hospital care for both cohorts tends to be regarded negatively, with the TCT units being the exception in most cases. Although for some, the specialist unit would have been their preferred place of death, it was not always an option perhaps because of lack of beds or geographical distance from the family home. However, the more generally unenthusiastic response to hospital care suggests there is much work to be done in making hospital palliative and end of life care a more acceptable option. Communication and good relationships between specialist services where there is an understanding of the child's needs and locally based more general services, seem central to a satisfactory experience – whether this is founded on shared care, reciprocal training opportunities or simply making contact before a crisis.

For the families of the children with complex life-limiting conditions, it may be difficult to predict when the end of their child's life will occur, and supportive care may move seamlessly into end of life care without being recognised. However, once a TYA with cancer has run out of treatment options and end of life appears inevitable, it may still be difficult to predict how long they will survive. Thus, both cohorts of parents may be faced with uncertainty that makes planning problematic. To introduce end of life care services too soon can be distressing for all concerned, yet not to have them planned well enough in advance can result in a crisis at a critical moment. It seems that for both cohorts early discussion between all parties about what the young person's preferences are can prepare the ground, yet this is reliant on an open awareness context that may not be adopted by some families.

There may be assumptions about how 'easy' (or difficult) or appropriate it is to communicate with the child or young person about the likelihood of their death, depending on their age and cognitive ability. Yet we have seen that no such assumptions can be made; the models of good practice based on honesty and open awareness may be no less difficult to implement with the TYAs with cancer than they are with much younger children or with young people who have cognitive impairments. Thus, the careful preparation and forward planning necessary in preparing for end of life care needs to be extended to dialogue about how and when the child or young person should be included in such a discussion, whatever their age or illness. One area of research that needs to be developed is how and when to talk about end of life care with children who have both cognitive impairments and a life-limiting illness.

The issue of choice is common to both cohorts – the choices to be made may be different but the need for options to be clear, and for parents to feel some sense of agency and empowerment, is significant. Clear information is necessary, based on forward planning, good communication between services and listening to what individual patients and their families need in their particular circumstances.

The emotional impact and support needs of the two cohorts are similar, because the distress they feel at the prospect of the death of a son or daughter is very much the same. The shock for the parents of the children with complex life-limiting conditions has usually come at birth, whereas the shock for the parents of the TYAs occurs unexpectedly during adolescence: but the emotional impact of facing the death of their son or daughter, despite all the differences, is very similar. Their requirements in preparing for the death and after bereavement may also be alike – but their needs are individual. Although the loss of a child is immense, as we have seen not all bereaved families follow a predictable model of grief and may need support of different types at different times.

Funding and the future

At the time of the Vickers et al. (2007) study into paediatric palliative care services for children with cancer in the UK, tertiary oncology services were commissioned regionally. As these authors say, if the provision of palliative care is included in oncology services, no distinction is made between home-based care and hospital care thus avoiding penalties for home-based care and enabling the provision of flexible palliative care services for children with cancer. For illnesses other than cancer, the funding of services for children with palliative care needs has been ad hoc and reliant on short-term injections of cash (DH 2007: 36). Funding varies widely across England and, according to the DH, there is not enough funding to provide the range of services specified in the ACT Care Pathway:

> Statutory funding from the NHS and Local Authority Children's Services (LACS) is the most sustainable funding, but too many key services are reliant on short-term grants or voluntary provision.
> (DH 2007: 5)

This document suggests that the funding priority should be community-based teams and that most services should be delivered jointly by health and social care involving both the NHS and LACS. There is a suggestion that paediatric palliative care teams can reduce the reliance on hospital services, making savings that will fund the team. Given what we have seen in this book about the lack of home-based and community services in some areas, and some parents' and patients' preferences for home-based care, 4 years after the publication of this DH report it is regrettable that community-based services are not more uniformly resourced across the country. In relation to the funding of hospice care, the discrepancy between adult and paediatric services is summed up as follows:

> Although adult hospices differ from children's hospices, they do provide a comparator in terms of statutory funding and in commissioning of end of life care. Although many adult hospices also face problems through lack of sustainable funding, in 2000 NHS funding for adult hospices averaged 28%. By 2004, this had increased to 38%, mostly as a result of the extra £50 m per annum made available for adults under the Cancer Plan. This extra £50 m is now recurrent in PCT baseline allocations ensuring it is available on a long-term basis for palliative/end of life care. There is therefore a sharp contrast between the funding and priority given to hospice services for adults and for children.
> (DH 2007: 35)

With regard to the young people in transition between paediatric and adult services who, as we have seen can fall through a gap between the two, Marsh et al. (2011) make the following recommendation:

> **Our conclusion overall is that young people should have the choice to stay with the relationships they have, adapted to age and changing need, and their support needs require creative joint funding under their and their families' control, possibly from a new national 'pot'.**
> (Marsh et al. 2011: 8, original emphasis)

At the time of writing, the organisation of health services in the UK was undergoing significant restructuring with the disbanding of PCTs and the transfer of responsibility for NHS commissioning to groups of GPs (Norridge 2011). We saw in Liz's comment at the start of this chapter that decisions on the allocation of care made by PCTs have been inconsistent and 'a huge postcode lottery' - it is to be hoped that any change in the funding structure will remedy the patchiness of provision rather than making it even more reliant on local priorities. The impact of the move from PCT to GP commissioning cannot yet be judged, but mention of end of life care by the House of Commons Health Committee is confined to two paragraphs (157 and 169) of their policy document on commissioning:

> Where service integration and continuity of care is important to secure the best clinical outcomes, patient experience and value for money (for example, in end of life care), the intention is that commissioners will be able to go to competitive tender and offer the service to one provider or 'prime contractor'.
> (House of Commons Health Committee 2011: 35-36)

and

> A crucial part of effective commissioning is the ability to assemble stable and coherent pathways of care, with all their constituent elements

seamlessly integrated. Such an approach is generally held to facilitate both the best outcomes for patients and value for money. It is particularly important where patients require complex, integrated packages of care, such as care for frail older people with multiple co-morbidities and end of life care.

(House of Commons Health Committee 2011: 38)

No mention is made in this document of palliative and end of life care specifically for children and young people, and a scan of other policy documents on the relevant NHS (2011) website revealed that many made no mention of palliative or end of life care. An interview with Clare, a senior care provider in the children's hospice movement, indicated that she thought end of life care for young people was a very low priority for the restructured services – indeed, she said 'I think we are like a flea on the end of a dog's tail'. Having tried to have a dialogue with the local GP Consortia, Clare told me that they 'politely' responded by saying 'We need to get our house in order first'. Thus, it seems that there are still many uncertainties about how services will be funded and what the priorities will be.

These funding issues relate to the UK; other countries in Europe, North America and elsewhere will have different funding streams and differently structured health care delivery. The research on which this book has been based cannot claim to be international, nor can it offer any systematic cross-cultural comparisons of policy and provision. Nevertheless, the inclusion of international literature and interviews with a limited number of non-UK participants from Australia, Canada, Germany and the USA, indicates that the participant families describe issues, challenges and dilemmas that have much in common and cross national boundaries. This book offers in-depth personal accounts of what it is like to care for a child who is dying; now we know what the issues are, what is needed is a quantitative, statistical study that maps provision across countries so that the expressed needs and concerns of those whose voices are represented in this book, and others who come after them, can have their needs met.

Appendix: Methodology

This book is based on findings from two studies. The first study explored the palliative and end of life care options for TYAs with cancer, and the second study was an evaluation of children's hospice services. The methods used in these two studies are considered separately.

Research into palliative and end of life care provision for TYAs with cancer

This part of the study used a mixed method approach of qualitative research interviews and service evaluation questionnaires and interviews. The qualitative research data are drawn from interviews with some 43 participants: hospice staff, and bereaved parents and family members. Hospice staff participants were recruited by approaching a selected sample of nine hospices, to ensure that children's, adolescent and adult hospice provision were included. Of the 21 professionals interviewed, some also had wider roles in the hospice movement and were thus able to offer an overview of the issues.

A number of parents and some siblings from bereaved families also participated. Most of these parents were introduced to me by staff at the hospices where I had been undertaking interviews, and some were introduced to me by the Teenage Cancer Trust. This part of the research included families whose children had died in a variety of care settings. As well as undertaking individual interviews with parents, some interviews were undertaken with couples and some with the whole family. I was also invited to observe and record a bereavement support group run by the Teenage Cancer Trust. This was not a focus group set up for my benefit, but a meeting of a group that met regularly, at which I asked no questions thus the issues, topics and discussion were spontaneous and my presence did not appear to influence the group's exchanges. In total, 22 interviews were undertaken with bereaved parents individually and 14 parents and family members participated in the bereavement support group.

All participants were offered the chance to select a pseudonym, but most preferred that their own first names should be used. The result is a mix of real names and pseudonyms in this text, so only the participants will be able to identify their own contribution. The use of genuine names can appear to be in contravention of codes of ethical conduct, and I have written on this topic elsewhere (Grinyer 2002b). However, as my approach with the participants in all aspects of this study

Palliative and End of Life Care for Children and Young People: Home, Hospice and Hospital, First Edition. Anne Grinyer.
© 2012 John Wiley & Sons, Ltd. Published 2012 by John Wiley & Sons, Ltd.

was that they should lead the process, I respected their wish to retain 'ownership' of their stories through the use of their real names if they wished. All interviews were audio-recorded with consent and subsequently transcribed verbatim.

Many of the interviews were face-to-face, those with hospice staff took place on the hospice premises, apart from one which took place in the hotel where I was staying. The face-to-face interviews with families took place in their homes apart from one, which again took place in the hotel where I was staying. Some interviews were undertaken by telephone as participants were scattered across the country and the project did not have the resources to allow for travel to each location (Thomas and Purdon 1994). However, I was unable to discern any substantial impact on the quality of the resulting interview data, which are rich and detailed, the phone conversations, usually lasting for at least as long as any of the face-to-face interviews, were also audio-recorded with consent. All participants were provided with information sheets, signed consent forms and were informed of their right to withdraw at any time without giving a reason. Consent for the use of the data for the purposes of publication was given by each participant.

The data were collected through qualitative interviews that adopted a grounded theory approach (Glaser and Strauss 1967), thus as new issues were raised by participants they were fed into subsequent interviews. However, I also gave the participants the opportunity to discuss their experience in an unstructured way to ensure that issues of significance to them had a chance of being raised. In this part of the study all interviews were conducted by me.

The qualitative interviews in this part of the study were done in conjunction with a service evaluation questionnaire in an attempt to map services for TYAs. The questionnaire was distributed to all the Teenage Cancer Trust units (nine at that time) and to selected NHS paediatric wards. After the main data collection period had finished, I became involved with the Teenage Cancer Trust evaluation of their palliative and end of life care services at their hospital-based units, which provided the opportunity to access additional data, which the TCT were generous enough to allow me to incorporate into this book. In this instance I did not collect the material myself but site visits were made to seven units by a trusted fieldworker (Zephyrine Barbarachild) who undertook observation, questionnaires and interviews that became the basis for a report we prepared for the TCT (Grinyer and Barbarachild 2011). A total of 23 interviews and 23 questionnaires were undertaken with staff whose roles are specified in the 'Participants' section of this book. Visits to the units also gave the researcher an opportunity to absorb the atmosphere and ethos of the care setting and use some observational methods. Informal discussions with staff during visits to the units have also provided valuable background information and understanding of the issues and challenges of offering appropriate end of life care for the age group. The data from this service evaluation have been used to enhance the research and other evaluation data, and have been instrumental particularly in considering 'training needs' and 'best practice' in the final chapter.

Data were collected until saturation was reached. Glaser and Strauss (1967) refer to this process as 'theoretical saturation': the point at which observations no longer serve to question or modify theories generated from earlier data (May 1997: 144). In order to make such a judgement, the collection of qualitative data incorporates a process of ongoing analysis throughout the data collection period (Robson 1995). New issues raised by a participant can be incorporated into subsequent interviews, so although such topics are generated in the first instance by the interviewee(s), the researcher can use them as the basis for a topic guide for future interviews. According to Pope and Mays (1996: 70), this process of ongoing thematic analysis often includes anticipated themes, and this was indeed the case.

However, they also point out that other issues arise during the fieldwork, and the thematic analysis can be used to develop taxonomies and express connections between the themes.

Although the researcher is constantly developing an analytical framework throughout the process, it is nevertheless crucial that analytical transparency and rigour are demonstrated if qualitative data are to avoid being dismissed as 'merely anecdotal' or highly selective. Mindful of such a requirement, the data were rigorously analysed using methods of data reduction, display and conclusion drawing (Miles and Huberman 1994). Miles and Huberman note that extended text is dispersed, poorly structured and extremely bulky, and that in order to avoid jumping to unfounded conclusions, or overweighting a particularly dramatic passage, certain processes must be observed during analysis. To this end, the data have been subjected to codification. They have been sorted and sifted in a manner that facilitates the identification of similar phrases, themes and patterns. Through the identification of commonalities and differences, and a consideration of the relationship between the variables, a set of generalisations was gradually developed to cover the consistencies discerned in the database.

Evaluation of children's hospice services

This part of the study was conducted separately; I was one of a team working on the service evaluation with Professor Sheila Payne and Zephyrine Barbarachild. The evaluation was commissioned by a children's hospice whose senior management team wished to understand how their services were experienced by users, and why some families and young people entitled to use the services had declined them. The evaluation used a mixed method approach of questionnaires followed up by interviews. The hospice approached participants on their database, and no attempt was made by the researcher to contact the hospice users until the recipients of the initial contact had agreed to participate. Service evaluation questionnaires were sent to the 76 parents and guardians of young people using the services of the children's hospice, and the recipients were invited to volunteer for follow-up interviews. This generated a 34% response rate of 26 completed questionnaires, and subsequent interviews with 11 families, eventually producing 24 interview participants who comprised of: three patients, three siblings, ten mothers, three fathers, two grandmothers, one paid carer, one bereaved mother and one bereaved sibling. These interviews were also conducted by Zephyrine Barbarachild, thus ensuring some continuity of approach with the data she collected for the TCT service evaluation (see above).

The data from the questionnaires yielded little in the way of relevant data to answer the central question but acted as a useful means to recruit to the qualitative part of the study. The questionnaire data were analysed by a statistician but the outcome has not been utilised in this book. The subsequent interviews with the questionnaire respondents were undertaken by Zephyrine in the families' homes and, although in contrast to the majority of the research discussed above I did not collect the data myself, I nevertheless had access to the recordings and fully transcribed interviews. Zephyrine also provided me with detailed field notes describing the family, their circumstances and home setting, which gave me a very clear picture of the context. I also had several meetings with Zephyrine during the analysis of the data, when she was able to fill in many details and make observations that were useful to my understanding of the families and their situations.

All participants were provided with information sheets and signed consent forms, and were informed of their right to withdraw without giving a reason. Consent for the use of the data from the hospice service evaluation for the purposes of publication was given by each participant, and the chief executive of the hospice in question also gave consent for the data to be used for this book. The details of the participants in this part of the study are included in a separate chart in the 'Participants' section of this book; in this case all participants from this evaluation have been allocated a pseudonym.

Case studies

I have used a case study approach in the presentation of some of the data both from the service evaluation and the TYA research. I have used the hospice that formed part of the service evaluation as the case study of a single institution to examine the issues that arise for users and I have selected a number of case studies of individuals as illustrations that exemplify the wider issues in the data. Case studies can be used in order to allow for the examination of detail missing in other methods (Gilbert 2008). There is no simple taxonomy within which various kinds of case study might be classified; they can be written for different purposes and at different analytical levels (Lincoln and Guba 1985). Lincoln and Guba (1985: 218-19) suggest that when sampling is done 'purposively' as in this instance, alternative criteria are necessary to ensure of the 'trustworthiness' of the method. These criteria are that: in place of internal validity there should be 'credibility', in place of external validity there should be 'transferability'; in place of reliability there should be 'dependability' and in place of objectivity there should be 'confirmability'. Although it may be difficult to verify that such safeguards to trustworthiness have been built in to the data collection and analysis, the accounts are consistent enough both on an individual and a collective basis that the trustworthiness of the data seems persuasive.

Ethics

Ethical approval was obtained from Lancaster University's Research Ethics Committee (UREC). Although the research study into end of life care for TYAs with cancer was approved by Lancaster University, additional approval was granted at individual hospices by their own ethics committees. The process varied at each hospice but providing the documentation approved by my university assisted in the hospice committees' decision making, and in no instance was I refused access. All participants were provided with information sheets and consent forms. The bereaved parents were approached by hospice staff initially and I approached them with sensitivity, given the nature of the interview that focused on the end of life care received by their son or daughter. On several occasions a parent became upset and I offered to suspend or terminate the interview, but in all cases the participant wished to continue as it was important to them that their account was fully heard. In each case I was prepared to offer information on sources of support if they were needed. All participants were fully informed about the nature and purpose of the research and about who would have access to the data. They were informed of their right to withdraw at any time without giving a reason and gave consent for their data to be used for publication. Indeed, they were particularly keen that their data should contribute to this book so that others would learn and benefit from their experience.

Although it is not necessary to have ethics committee approval for a service evaluation, those undertaken in the NHS still have to be approved through the research governance process, and local consent at each site needs to be granted. This process was undertaken for the TYA study. As in this part of the study the service evaluation applied only to approaching health professionals in order to map service provision, additional ethical approval was not sought. In contrast, the service evaluation of the children's hospice involved collecting data from service users – the patients (where appropriate) and their families. As the nature of this investigation seemed to raise all the same issues as if the enquiry had been 'research', additional ethics committee approval was sought. As this hospice service evaluation did not come under the jurisdiction of the NHS, consent was sought through UREC and was granted. All the same ethical considerations given to the research with the parents in the TYA study were afforded to the parents and families in the service evaluation.

There could be a danger that service evaluation can be used as a 'back door' method to undertake research without the need to undergo rigorous ethical approval. As APCRC (2010) state:

It can be difficult to distinguish some types of evaluation from research, since like research, evaluation:

- May provide cost and/or benefit information on a service
- Use quantitative and qualitative data to explore activities and issues
- May identify strengths and weaknesses of services
- Evaluation may also include elements of research e.g. collecting additional data or changes to choices of treatment

Both research and evaluation involves addressing clearly defined questions using systematic and rigorous methods. However, the key difference is that research aims to derive generalisable new knowledge, but evaluation does not. Service evaluation is performed to meet specific local needs and generalising the results to other settings is not part of the design of the project.
(APCRC 2010)

Such a definition could be problematic, given that a service evaluation like my own among the TCT units derives data from a variety of locations. After mapping provision for the age group across a variety of locations in the UK, it is difficult to not make an onward connection about how the provision across the country is experienced. Thus, it seems that the requirement that service evaluation should not derive generalisable new knowledge creates an artificial constraint. Although the purpose of the evaluation may not be to achieve such an aim, it would seem perverse not to benefit from the outcome if such data were produced. However, mindful of the danger of using such an approach inappropriately, ethical approval was sought for the service evaluation of the children's hospice, thus presumably freeing the data to be used for something more akin to research purposes.

It is crucial that all research, but particularly in such a sensitive field, is conducted ethically and with proper regard for the wellbeing of the participants. Ethics committee scrutiny and approval is one way of ensuring that this process is rigorously governed and that studies are properly designed, but it is the point of contact and interaction between the participants and the researcher/interviewer that will shape the experience for the participant. In the case of both the TYA research and the hospice service evaluation, the researchers (Zephyrine and myself) had extensive experience of undertaking difficult and sensitive interviews with people who could be regarded as vulnerable. However, those who are vulnerable should not be precluded from participating: where the interviewer uses a sensitive approach, the interviewee can find the experiencing empowering, feeling that their stories, views and experiences are being 'heard' and that they are contributing knowledge that may make a difference. As Contro et al. (2002) report, the families who participated in their study on paediatric end of life care all expressed gratitude at being given the opportunity to tell their stories and contribute to the improvement of services.

Although the formal data collection methods have been described in this account, I have also absorbed a considerable amount of additional information that contextualises and informs many of my observations in this book, while spending 2 years immersed in the field of palliative and end of life care services for children and young adults, making a number of visits of several days' duration to hospitals and hospices, and talking 'off the record' to a wide variety of interested parties, both users and professionals. Such material does not constitute formally collected data and its status is ambiguous, but it cannot be disregarded. I have written elsewhere about the status of data observed informally in the field of interest and the legitimacy of using it (Grinyer 2001). Suffice it to say here that I have only quoted from data for which I have explicit consent and any additional observations have been generalised, in order to respect the boundaries between the material that has specific consent for use in publications and that which does not. Nevertheless, readers should be aware that a wider knowledge informs this work than that which is formally accounted for.

References

ACT (2009) *A guide to the development of children's palliative care services*, 3rd edn. Association of Children's Palliative Care, Bristol.

ACT (2011a) *A Care Pathway to Support Extubation within a Children's Palliative Care Framework*, retrieved from: http://www.act.org.uk/page.asp?section=406&sectionTitle=A+care+pathway+to+support+extubation+within+a+children%27s+palliative+care+framework, 7.4.11.

ACT (2011b) *A parent's guide: Making critical care choices for your child*, retrieved from: http://www.act.org.uk/page.asp?section=406&sectionTitle=A+care+pathway+to+support+extubation+within+a+children%27s+palliative+care+framework, 7.4.11.

ACT (2011c) *Children's Palliative Care Handbook for GPs*, retrieved from: http://www.act.org.uk/page.asp?section=411&sectionTitle=Children%27s+palliative+care+handbook+for+GPs 11.5.11.

ACT (2011d) Press Release: *ACT launches essential symptom management handbook to support children with life-limiting conditions*, Issued 13.6.11.

Alderson, P. (1992) In the genes or in the stars? Children's competence to consent, *Journal of Medical Ethics*, Vol. 18 (3) 119–124.

APCRC (Avon Primary Care Research Collaborative) NHS Bristol (2010) What is Service Evaluation? retrieved from: http://www.apcrc.nhs.uk/Service_Evaluation/what_is_service_evaluation.htm#6, 23.4.10.

Apter, T. (2001) *The Myth of Maturity: What Teenagers Need from Parents to Become Adults*, W.W. Norton and Co Inc, New York.

Arbuckle, J., Cotton, R., Eden, T.O.B., Jones, R. and Leonard, R. (2005) Who Should Care for Young People with Cancer? *Cancer and the Adolescent*, (eds T.O.B Eden, R.D. Barr, A. Bleyer and M. Whiteson) pp. 231–240, Blackwell, Oxford.

Ashby, M.A., Kosky, R.J., Laver, H.T. and Sims, E.B. (1991) An enquiry into death and dying at the Adelaide Children's Hospital: a useful model? *Medical Journal of Australia*. Vol. 154 (3), 165–170.

Association of Children's Palliative Care (2007) *The Transition Care Pathway*, Bristol, ACT, http://www.endoflifecareforadults.nhs.uk/eolc/files/ACT-Transition_care_pathway_Apr2007.pdf.

Baker McCall, J. (2004) *Bereavement Counselling: Pastoral Care for Complicated Grieving*, The Haworth Press, Binghampton.

Benini, F., Spizzichino, M., Trapanotto M. and Ferrante, A. (2008) Pediatric palliative care, *Italian Journal of Pediatrics*. Retrieved from: http://www.ncbi.nlm.nih.gov/pmc/articles/PMC2687538/34: 9.9.10.

Berzoff, J. and Silverman, P.R. (eds) (2004) *Living with Dying*, Columbia University Press, New York.

Brannen, J., Dodd, K., Oakley, A. and Storey, P. (1994) *Young People, Health and Family Life*, Open University Press, Buckingham.

Brook, L, Vickers, J. and Barber, M. (2006) Place of Care. In: *Oxford Textbook of Palliative Care for Children*, (eds A. Goldman, R. Hain and S. Liben) pp. 533–548, Oxford University Press, Oxford.

Brown, E. (2006) Ritual and Religion. In: *Oxford Textbook of Palliative Care for Children*, (eds. A. Goldman, R. Hain and S. Liben) pp. 204–227, Oxford University Press, Oxford.

Brown, E. with Warr, B. (2007) *Supporting the Child and the Family in Paediatric Palliative Care*, Jessica Kingsley, London.

CCLG (Children's Cancer and Leukaemia Group) (2007) *Choices: when it seems there are none*, CCLG, Leicester.

CHANGE Cancer Series Accessible Book 3 (2010a) *Palliative Care, End of Life Care and Bereavement*, CHANGE, Leeds.

CHANGE Cancer Series Carers Book 3 (2010b) *Palliative Care, End of Life Care and Bereavement*, CHANGE, Leeds.

Clark, D. and Wright, M. (2003) *Transitions in End of Life Care: Hospice and Related Developments in Eastern Europe and Central Asia*, Open University Press, Buckingham.

CLIC Sargent (2006) *When There is no Longer a Cure*, CLC Sargent, London.

Contro, N., Larson, J., Scofield, S., Sourkes, B. and Cohen, H.J. (2002) Family perspectives on the quality of pediatric palliative care, *Archives of Pediatric and Adolescent Medicine*, Vol. 156 (1), 14–19.

Contro, N. and Scofield, S. (2006) The Power of their Voices: Child and Family Assessment in Pediatric Palliative Care. In: *Oxford Textbook of Palliative Care for Children*, (eds A. Goldman, R. Hain and S. Liben) pp. 143–153, Oxford University Press, Oxford.

Contro, N.A., Larson, J., Scofield, S., Sourkes, B. and Cohen, H.J. (2004) Hospital staff and family perspectives regarding quality of pediatric palliative care, *Pediatrics*, Vol. 114 (5), 1248-1252.

Craig, F. (2006) Adolescents and Young Adults. In: *Oxford Textbook of Palliative Care for Children*, (eds A. Goldman, R. Hain and S. Liben) pp. 108–118, Oxford University Press, Oxford.

Darnill, S. and Gamage, B. (2006) The patient's journey: palliative care – a parent's view, *British Medical Journal*, 332, 1494-1495.

Davis, R. (2009) Caring for the Child at the End of Life. In: *Palliative Care for Children and Families: An Interdisciplinary Approach*, (eds J. Price and P. McNeilly), pp. 172–191, Palgrave Macmillan, Basingstoke.

Department of Health (2007*) Palliative care services for children and young people in England*, retrieved from: http://palliativecarefunding.org.uk/wp-content/uploads/2010/08/Palliative-Care-For-C+YP-in-England.pdf, 18.4.11.

Department of Health (2008) *Better Care: Better Lives – Improving Outcomes and Experiences for Children, Young People and Their Families Living with Life-Limiting and Life-Threatening Conditions*, retrieved from: http://www.dh.gov.uk/en/Publicationsandstatistics/Publications/PublicationsPolicyAnd Guidance/DH_083106, 14.2.10.

Dominica (1987) The role of the hospice for the dying child, *British Journal of Hospital Medicine*, October 1987, pp. 334-343.

Drake, R., Frost, J. and Collins, J.J. (2003) The symptoms of dying children, *Journal of Pain and Symptom Management*. Vol. 26 (1), 594-603.

Dussel, V., Kreicbergs, U., Hilden, J.M., Watterson, J., Moore, C., Turner, B.G., Weeks, J.C. and Wolfe, J. (2009) Looking beyond where children die: determinants and effects of planning a child's location of death, *Journal of Pain Symptom Management.* Vol. 37 (1), 33-43.

EAPC (2009) *Palliative Care for Infants, Children and Young People*, retrieved from: http://www.eapcnet.org/download/forTaskforces/Paediatric/PC-FACT. pdf, 14.2.10.

Engel, M. (2005) The Day the Sky Fell in, *Guardian Colour Supplement*, 3.12.05: pp. 18-26.

Eysenbach, G. (2001) What is e-health? *Journal of Medical Internet Research*, Vol. 3(2), retrieved from http://www.jmir.org/2001/2/e20/, 1.4.10.

Feudtner, C., DiGuiseppe, D.L. and Neff, J.M. (2003) Hospital care for children and young adults in the last year of life: a population based study, *BMC Medicine*, 1(3) retrieved from http://www.biomedcentral.com/1741-7015/1/3/, 5.4.11.

Feudtner, C., Feinstein, J.A., Satchell, M., Zhao, H. and Kang, T.I. (2007) Shifting place of death among children with complex chronic conditions in the United States, 1989-2003, *Journal of the American Medical Association*, Vol. 297 (24), 2725-2732.

Feudtner, C., Silveria, M.J. and Christakis, D.A. (2002) Where do children with complex chronic conditions die? Patterns in Washington State, 1980-1998, *Pediatrics*, Vol. 109 (4), 656-660.

Field, M.J. and Behrman, R.E. (eds) (2003) *When Children Die*, Institute of Medicine (IOM), The National Academies Press, Washington.

Freyer, D.R. (2004) Care of the dying adolescent: special considerations, *Pediatrics* Vol. 113 (2), 381-388.

George, R. and Hutton, S. (2003) Palliative care in adolescents, *European Journal of Cancer*, Vol. 39 (18), 2662-2668.

Gilbert, N. (2008) Research, Theory and Method. In: *Researching Social Life* (ed. N. Gilbert) 3rd edn. pp. 21-40, Sage, London,

Glaser, B. and Strauss, A. (1967) *The Discovery of Grounded Theory*, Aldine, Chicago.

Grant, S. (2005). *Standing on His Own Two Feet*, Jessica Kingsley, London.

Grinyer, A. (2001) Ethical dilemmas in non-clinical health research, *Nursing Ethics*, Vol. 8 (2), 123-132.

Grinyer, A. (2002a) *Cancer in Young Adults: Through Parents' Eyes*, Open University Press, Buckingham.

Grinyer, A. (2002b) The Anonymity of Research Participants: Assumptions, Ethics and Practicalities, *Social Research Update, Issue 36*, University of Surrey.

Grinyer, A. (2004) Young adults with cancer: parents' interaction with health care professionals, *The European Journal of Cancer Care*, Vol. 13, 88-95.

Grinyer, A. (2006) Caring for a young adult with cancer: the impact on mothers' health, *Health and Social Care in the Community*, Vol. 14 (4), 311-318.

Grinyer, A. (2007a) *Young People Living with Cancer: implications for policy and practice*, Open University Press, Buckingham.

Grinyer, A. (2007b) The biographical impact of teenage and adolescent cancer, *Chronic Illness*, Vol. 3 (4), 265-277.

Grinyer, A. (2009) Contrasting parental perspectives with those of teenagers and young adults with cancer: comparing the findings from two qualitative studies, *European Journal of Oncology Nursing*, Vol. 13, 192-198.

Grinyer, A. and Barbarachild. Z. (2011) *Teenage and young adult palliative and end of life care service evaluation*, Report, Teenage Cancer Trust, London.

Grinyer, A., Payne, S. and Barbarachild, Z. (2010) Issues of power, control and choice in children's hospice respite care services: a qualitative study, *International Journal of Palliative Nursing*, Vol. 14 (5), 505-510.

Grinyer, A. and Thomas, C. (2004) The importance of place of death in young adults with terminal cancer, *Mortality*, Vol. 9 (2), 114-131.

Higginson, I. and Thompson, M. (2003) Children and young people who die from cancer: epidemiology and place of death in England (1995–9), *British Medical Journal*, Vol. 327, 478–9.

Hinds, P.S., Drew, D., Oakes, L.L., Fouladi, M., Spunt, S.L., Church, C. and Furman, W. (2005) End-of life-care preferences of pediatric patients with cancer, *Journal of Clinical Oncology*, Vol. 23 (36), 9146–9154.

House of Commons Health Committee (2011) *Commissioning: Further issues*, Vol. 1, retrieved from: http://www.publications.parliament.uk/pa/cm201011/cmselect/cmhealth/796/796i.pdf, 17.4.11.

Hynson, J.L. (2006) The Child's Journey: Transition from Health to Ill Health. In: *Oxford Textbook of Palliative Care for Children* (eds A. Goldman, R. Hain, and S. Liben) pp. 14–27, Oxford University Press, Oxford.

Kelly, D. and Gibson F. (eds) (2008), *Cancer Care for Adolescents and Young Adults*, Blackwell, Oxford.

Kirsti A. and Dyer M.D. (2006), *What are End of Life and End of Life Care?* Retrieved from: http://dying.about.com/od/hospicecare/f/endoflife.htm, 25.4.10

Kushnik, H.L. (2010) Trusting them with the truth – disclosure and the good death for children with terminal illness, *Virtual Mentor*, Vol. 12 (7), 573–577.

Lenton, S., Goldman, A., Eaton, N. and Southall, D. (2006) Development and Epidemiology. In: *Oxford Textbook of Palliative Care for Children* (eds A. Goldman, R. Hain and S. Liben) pp. 3–13, Oxford University Press, Oxford.

Lewis, I. (2005) Patterns of Care for Teenagers and Young Adults with Cancer: is there a single blueprint of care? *Cancer and the Adolescent* (eds T.O.B Eden, R.D. Barr, A. Bleyer and M. Whiteson) pp. 241–258, Blackwell Oxford.

Lewis, M. and Prescott, H. (2006) Impact of Life-Limiting Illness on the Family. In: *Oxford Textbook of Palliative Care for Children* (eds A. Goldman, R. Hain and S. Liben) pp. 154–178, Oxford University Press, Oxford.

Lincoln, Y.S. and Guba, E.G. (1985) *Naturalistic Inquiry*, Sage, London.

Marsh, S., Cameron, M., Duggan, M. and Rodrigues, J. (with Eisenstadt, N., Iskander, R. and Stone, J.) (2011) *Young people with life limiting conditions: transition to adulthood*, Public Service Works retrieved from: http://www.publicserviceworks.com/userdocs/report%20v3%20for%20MCCCfull%20final.pdf, 20.6.11.

May, T. (1997) *Social Research: Issues, Methods and Process*, Open University Press, Buckingham.

McCallum, D.E., Byrne, P. and Bruera, E. (2000) *Journal of Pain and Symptom Management* Vol. 20 (6), 417–423.

Macdonald, M.E., Liben, S., Carnevale, F.A., Rennick, J.E., Wolf, S.L., Meloche, D. and Cohen, S.R. (2005) Parental perspectives on hospital staff members' acts of kindness and commemoration after a child's death, *Pediatrics* Vol. 116 (4), 884–890.

Meyer D.K., Ratichek, S., Berhe, H., Stewart, S., McTavish, F., Gustafson, D. and Parsons, S.K. (2010) Development of a health-related website for parents of children receiving hematopoietic stem cell transplant: HSCT-CHESS, *Journal of Cancer Survivorship: Research and Practice*, Vol. 4 (1), 67–73.

Miles, M.B. and Huberman, A.M. (1994) *Qualitative Data Analysis*, Sage, London.

Milo, E.M. (1997) Maternal responses to the life and death of a child with a developmental disability: a story of hope, *Death Studies*, Vol. 21 (5), 443–76.

Montel, S., Laurence, V., Copel, L., Paquement, H. and Flahault, C. (2009) Place of death of adolescents and young adults with cancer: first study in a French population, *Palliative and Supportive Care*, 7, 27–35.

National Cancer Intelligence Network (NCIN) (2011) *Place of death for children, teenagers and young adults with cancer in England*, NCIN Data Briefing, www.ncin.org.uk/databriefings

NHS (2011) *NHS Evidence - Commissioning*, retrieved from: http://www.library.nhs.uk/commissioning/SearchResults.aspx?searchText=%22gp+commissioning%22+OR+%22gp+commissioner%22+OR+%22gp+commissioners%22&tabID=290&, 17.4.11.

NHS National End of Life Care Programme (undated) retrieved from: http://www.endoflifecareforadults.nhs.uk/, 7.4.11. Policy Exchange, London.

Norridge, E. (2011) *Implementing GP Commissioning*, retrieved from:http://www.policyexchange.org.uk/images/publications/pdfs/Implementing_GP_Commissioning_-_Apr__11.pdf, 17.4.11.

Pope, C. and Mays, N. (1996) *Qualitative Research in Health Care*, Blackwell, Oxford.

Pfund, R. (2007) *Palliative Care Nursing of Children and Young People*, Radcliffe Publishing, Oxford.

Price, J. and McFarlane, M. (2009) Palliative Care for Children - a Unique Way of Caring. In: *Palliative Care for Children and Families: An Interdisciplinary Approach*, (eds J. Price and P. McNeilly), pp. 1-17, Palgrave Macmillan, Basingstoke:

Riches, G. and Dawson, P. (2000) *An Intimate Loneliness: Supporting Bereaved Parents and Siblings*, Open University Press, Buckingham.

Robson, C. (1995) *Real World Research*, Blackwell, Oxford.

Rosenblatt, P.C. (2000) *Parent Grief: Narratives of Loss and Relationship*, Taylor and Francis, Philadelphia.

Runswick-Cole, K. (2010) Living with dying and disablism: death and disabled children, *Disability & Society*, Vol. 25 (7), 813-826.

Sheetz, M.J. and Bowman, M.A (2008) Pediatric palliative care: an assessment of physicians' confidence in skill, desire for training, and willingness to refer for end-of-life care. *American Journal of Hospital Palliative Care*, Vol. 25 (2), 100-105.

Silverman, P.R. (2000) *Never too Young to Know: Death in Children's Lives*, Oxford University Press, Oxford.

Sourkes, B. (1977) Facilitating family coping with childhood cancer, *Journal of Pediatric Psychology*, Vol. 2 (2), 65-67.

Thomas, J. and Chalmers, A. (2009) Bereavement Care. In: *Palliative Care for Children and Families: An Interdisciplinary Approach*, (eds J. Price and P. McNeilly), pp. 192-212, Palgrave Macmillan, Basingstoke.

Thomas, R. and Purdon, S. (1994) Telephone Methods for Social Surveys, *Social Research Update*, Issue 8, University of Surrey.

Turkoski, B. (2003) A mother's orders: about truth telling, *Home Healthcare Nurse*, Vol. 21 (2), 81-83.

Vickers, J., Thompson, A., Collins, G.S., Childs, M. and Hain, R. (2007), Place and provision of palliative care for children with progressive cancer: a study by the paediatric oncology nurses' forum/united kingdom children's cancer study group palliative care working group, *Journal of Clinical Oncology*, Vol. 25 (28), 4472-4476.

Wiener, L., Ballard, E., Brennan, T., Battles, H., Martinez, P. and Pao, M. (2008) How I wish to be remembered: the use of an advance care planning document in adolescent and young adult populations, *Journal of Palliative Medicine*, Vol. 11 (120), 1309-1313.

Wolfe, J., Holcombe Grier, H.E., Klar, N., Levin, S.B., Ellenbogen, J.M., Salem-Schatz, S., Emanuel, E.J. and Weeks, J.C. (2000) Symptoms and suffering at the end of life in children with cancer, *The New England Journal of Medicine*, Vol. 342 (5), 326-333.

Woolfson, L. (2004) Family well-being and disabled children: A psychosocial model of disability-related child behaviour problems, *British Journal of Health Psychology* Vol. 9 (1), 1-13.

Index

Note: Page numbers in bold refers to tables.

Palliative and End of Life Care for Children and Young People: Home, Hospice
and Hospital, First Edition. Anne Grinyer.
© 2012 John Wiley & Sons, Ltd. Published 2012 by John Wiley & Sons, Ltd.